# Copyright MuscleSports.net

This book may not be copied in any way, shape or form, except for small excerpts for the purposes of promotion or reviews.

# Table of Contents:

# Introduction:

Bodybuilding is growing by leaps and bounds throughout the world today. It is the one sport where everyone is welcome. You don't have to be a certain height or weight, or even a boy or girl; everyone can do this and reap tremendous benefits. It gives the shy person a way to communicate and even helps bridge that shyness toward new friendships. Bodybuilding builds self-esteem, confidence and sense of pride in all those who truly love the sport.

Why I Wrote This Book

I wrote this book because I see allot of young beginning bodybuilders getting off on the wrong foot when it come to training, eating and the true bodybuilding life style. To many are caught up in a quick fix mentality that is destructive to everything they want as a bodybuilder. When I look around I see a void out in the public space where those who know are not are being passed over for the flash and glitz of a good story of how you can go from zero to hero in 12 months with the right drugs or other accessories. If you tried this approach you will burnout and eventually leave bodybuilding altogether or just hang around on the fringes. Bedrock was written to take your beginning body and transform you into a walking, talking, and extremely health bodybuilding athlete. We give you the workouts; nutritional guideline plus more to help you construct a bodybuilding foundation that can help you achieve anything in life.

Who Am I to Write This

I've been in the bodybuilding since 1978 when I first started lifting weight at McCellan AFB as a dependent. I have a BS degree in Computer Engineering, with minors in Mathematics and Health Science.  Since then I have trained 100's of competitors and non-competitor alike, who want to make their lives better. Presently I own many training and information website geared toward health and wellness. In writing this book I wanted to pack in the basic rules anyone starting out in bodybuilding should know and follow to help avoid pitfalls and actually lay a solid foundation for either competition or just exceptional health through out their life.

What You'll Find Here:

Gym Basics
Sample Routines
Dietary Guides
Sample Eating plans and Menus
Life Style Tips
Grocery Shopping List


**Darryl Lipscomb**
CEO DLI Digital Media
MuscleSports.net

# Chapter 1 Why?

## Why Write this Book?

Why did we want to write this book? I was asked that about a year ago when I began thinking of writing this book by someone who has written hard copy books and a few e-book like this one. I told him I was tired of seeing some of the stuff out there that says you can only get this far without taking some kind of drug, or some other forms of exotic pharmacology. Plus I had been seeing people giving advice on training that really doesn't make allot of sense. You have beginning bodybuilders and powerlifters doing routines that make you cringe. You see split routines for way more seasoned folk, training this body part in the morning and another one in the evening. Wearing lifting suits, wrapping knees, using straps and a host of other accessories just to move the weight.

## Why Bedrock Training?

Beginning bodybuilding is the most important time in you journey to build a complete physique and lay a foundation of strength. With all the information floating around out in the public sphere about training it can be a bit daunting to actually know where to begin. Some guides on social media would have you think that you can follow any kind of routine if you just ate the right foods or took the perfect drug cycle. This type of miss information can't be any farther from the true if it tried. Drugs alone will never get you to a great physique or a record breaking total. Proper training along with correct eating practices will greatly improve you chances of obtaining the body, strength and power you have wanted for so long. **Bedrock Training** principles are the fundamentals of bodybuilding and strength that builds a solid foundation of training and nutrition concepts that you will be able to build off of for your entire time in bodybuilding or other sports. This a challenging course that will take you from beginner to intermediate and then seasoned novice over the course of 104 weeks (that's 2 years). Real bodybuilding and strength training is not a quick fix but a consistent and steady climb up towards your goals of a strong, healthy, aesthetic physique fill with all the power and athleticism it can hold.

# Chapter 2 The Beginner

**Finding the Right Gym.**

Before you can get started on your bodybuilding journey you have to find the right training place for you. We have seen these people everyday, in every gym around the world. The come in and are immediately overwhelmed with why am I here, I don't like the music, these people are loud, and on, and on. It's not that this person doesn't want to workout it that they are not in the right environment. Being a bodybuilder requires being in a bodybuilding gym. It doesn't have to be as they say hardcore, but it does have to be a place where going through a hard training session won't garner stares and condemnation from fellow members and management. These place on;y want your money and should be avoided by the bodybuilder at all cost. We have 5 keys to finding the right gym for your bodybuilding purposes.

**<u>Top Five Things to Look For:</u>**

**1: Location** - Where's it located? To far means missed workout and bouts of procrastination. Find a place not so far that your dread driving there.

**2: Hours of Operation** - What hours are they open? Do these hours work for all possible schedules you may have?

**3: Cost of Membership** - Some places charge yearly dues on top of monthly fees. Some places only allow annual contracts. Make sure the amount and payment plans fit your budget and have no hidden cost for things you don't want or will not use.

**4: Cleanliness** - Inspect the equipment, is it kept clean and presentable. Are the locker rooms and facilities clean and sanitary? Remember your're going to be here with allot of other people and clean and safe environment is crucial to avoiding colds and sickness.

**5: Look at the Cliental** - For the bodybuilder this is one of the most important things you should observe. If you see others doing what it is you want to be doing then chances are they won't mind if your make faces or grunt a little when lifting something heavy.

**Extra Tip:** Check out your soon to be gym at least during 2 different time slots to make sure it fits your needs because workouts at quitting time (5PM-8PM) give you a very good indicator to the gyms financial stability, so as to not join some gym to only be left in the cold a few months down the road.

**What to Wear and What Not to Wear**

Now you would think this one would be very easy for almost everyone to get right, would you? Well you would be **WRONG**. In the past I have had guys show up for workouts in jeans, short shorts (we don't need to see that), smelling of liquor, and work uniforms. I have also had girls in high heels, tube tops, way to tight shorts, pajamas, sandals, and the list can go on for days about both sexes. Your gym attire should be loose but comfortable fitting clothing, and Rubber soled ankle supported Cross Trainer or mid top athletic shoes. The fabric of you clothing should be breathable because your going to sweat not see through. No mesh tops, string tank tops or any kinds of shirts that can and will get caught in equipment. Good shoes with quality ankle support, and with a flexible, sure grip rubber sole. Cross trainers tend to be the best fit, but some basketball shoes are very good also. Following these guidelines will let you focus on what your there for your workout, and not be adjusting yourself after every set or exercise.

**Gym Etiquette**

The first thing we are going to talk about is something that used to be taught in the oldschool days of the 60's, 70's, and even the early 80's when I learned to workout and its called Gym Etiquette. Gym etiquette is about you bowing or curtseying or eating with the right utensil. No gym etiquette is about how to use the gym for the very purpose its there for - Training. Do not enlist yourself in these top 10 misguided gym behaviors and you will not see you progress derailed as so many have.

**Top 10 Do's and Don't for Excellent Gym Etiquette:**

**Don't bring your Cell Phone on the Gym Floor -** Unless you're a critical professional like a on call doctor, fireman or police officer, you don't need your cell phone with you during your workout.

**Don't hog equipment** - Do your set or set in a timely fashion and move on to the next exercise. You're not the only one wanting to use the piece of equipment.

**Don't invade other personal space** - Others have the right to workout in peace, and with some one invading their personal space this id not possible. Show respect and ask to join in, pick the next exercise if possible or just wait until they are done. Your asking will usually get you on the equipment fast than you think.

**Let someone working in if possible** - Letting someone work in between sets is a good way for you to time your sets. It will also let others know that your serious about your workouts and sets precedent for future encounters.

**No posing or primping on the gym floor** - The gym floor is not a place for show or exhibitions. You're there to train and that it. Save the glamour stuff for another time, because this is not IT!

**Re-Rack Your Weights** - You took it off the rack so put it back where you got it form. Yeah we've all seen the videos of Professional bodybuilders dropping huge dumbbells on the floor after and intense set. The thing is they have people that shadow them during their workouts who do pick up the weights and re-rack them. Unless you got the money **RE-RACK YOUR WEIGHTS**!

**Don't drop your weights** - This goes along with the previous rule. Dropping weights is dangerous and can and has gotten many people injured. Always when possible put weight down in as controlled a manner as you possibly can. This saves you and others from injury. Just remember if your injured you can't train, and if you can't train you can't advanced your dreams.

**Keep it PG** - Keep your language under control at all times. Their may be times when you want to yell something but that is energy you should be putting toward your current or next set. Some of the loudest people you will hear in the gym are usually not those competing on the highest levels. They know it not about the attention but the work itself.

**Personal Hygiene** - This one is last but it one of the foremost ones that you need to address each and everyday. Wearing clean clothes and keeping great personal hygiene will open many doors for you that can not be explained in this one book. Good hygiene is also one of the quickest ways to improve your health and wellness.

Follow these Gym Etiquette tip and you will have a leg up on most people in everyday life and be well on your way to achieving the personal goals that you have set for your self.

## Bag of Tools

Every good bodybuilder carries him or her a gym bag filled with the essentials they need to get their workouts done and propel them on to whatever next in the day. As a newbie beginner you to need to have yourself a very well equipped gym bag so every thing you need is their for you when you need it. Since your level of need doesn't come up to that of a top level armature or professional your essentials should be limited to a few basic items. Over the years I have compiled a list of the items I have every trainee bring so we don't have interruptions to their training and all workout are completed with out fail.

**Change of fresh clothing** - Always bring a fresh shirt or pullover to replace the one you just sweated up. It helps keep the body warm as it begins to cool down after your training session. You may also need extra clothing if you intend to freshen up before leaving.

**Gym Towel** - This should be a no-brainer but you would be surprised how many people expect the facility to provide them with a towel. It's not the 1950's and hardly any club does that for free. Grab yourself a reasonable size towel that is of average size. It helps you by covering equipment to prevent germs and bacteria from affecting you. You're going to sweat so bring a towel.

**Weight lifting Belt** (Optional for first 6 months) - This is optional for most beginning bodybuilder because you should not be lifting anything of such weight that you need to protect you lumbar region. You will need to purchase a belt though as you progress through you first year to become accustomed to its fit and as weight and intensity of effort progresses after the first six months. Get a good solid weight lifting belt and not a back belt, which is a totally different piece of equipment.

**Weight lifting Chalk** (Optional for first 6 months) - Weight lifting chalk is one of the biggest bugaboos in the gym business. If when you are looking for a place to workout ask the person assisting you if they allow you to use chalk. Allot of newer gyms are kind of skittish in allowing chalk because they say it messy and hard to clean up, which is total crap. If they say yes then you're in a good place to conduct your training, if they say no ask why. Your going to need to rub a little chalk on your hands during the second six months because of sweat sometimes to get a good grip and prevent injury. Don't assume about chalk, its important always **ASK!**

**Water Bottle** - A good solid 32oz plus size water bottle is probably the best size to keep you well hydrated and refreshed going through your workout. Don't bring the gallon water jugs thinking that hardcore it just cheap and those jugs puncture easily. Get a thick clear, BPA free plastic bottle like the one recommended for long hiking trip, as those can be dropped hundreds of times and not crack of spill a drop

That's all you will need in your gym bag for your couple of years. You say what about lifting straps or something. This is something that truly pisses me off when I see people strapping up on every set from start to finish. It really makes no sense when the person doesn't have any credible amount of time in the gym under their belt. **During the first 2 years of your training you shouldn't ever touch a lifting strap, NOT FOR SHRUGS, DEADLIFTS, PULLDOWNS, BARBELL ROWS, DUMBBELL ROWS, T-BAR ROWS --- NOTHING!** One of the first things I was taught was if you couldn't pick it up or hold it on your own than the weights to heavy. The time for straps is far down the line right now it's about building a foundation of strength and grip strength is crucially important to build.

# Chapter 3 Concepts Training

## <u>Congratulations You Have Made a Wise Choice</u>

Choosing to start a bodybuilding lifestyle during your teenage years is probably one of the wisest choices a teenager could make for him or her self. This world is littered with allot people choosing the wrong paths early in life and finding out the mistakes they have made later in life. Choosing the bodybuilding life style can benefit you in every aspect of your life from sport, fitness, nutrition, self-esteem, physical health, intellect, and much, much more. Bodybuilding and strength training has lifted many a person out of poverty, jail, drugs, and many more pressures of life. Yes you have mad a very wise choice, a wise choice indeed.

## <u>What Old is New Again!</u>

When we begin training, as a new comer we want to do is gain muscle, and hell look damn good in the process. We get allot of questions, like how often do I workout and what exercises do I choose and how many time do I perform each movement. Do I workout 5-6-7 days a week? What do I eat to gain the most muscle mass? Do I have to take drugs to do this or are there more natural ways. These are all some very good question and we are going to try an answer each and every one of these and quite a few more you may not have thought of in this training manual for beginning bodybuilding. The purpose of this manual is to give you the foundations in training, nutrition, and life style so that after 2 years of following these principles you can with a little professional help began thinking about competition in your given athletic goals.


# <u>Lessons From the Past</u>

In today's bodybuilding world everyone believes the 3-day a week training schedule is one that is a relic of the past and its usefulness is also a thing of the past. The 3-day a week schedule is perhaps one of the most mass-producing natural bodybuilding 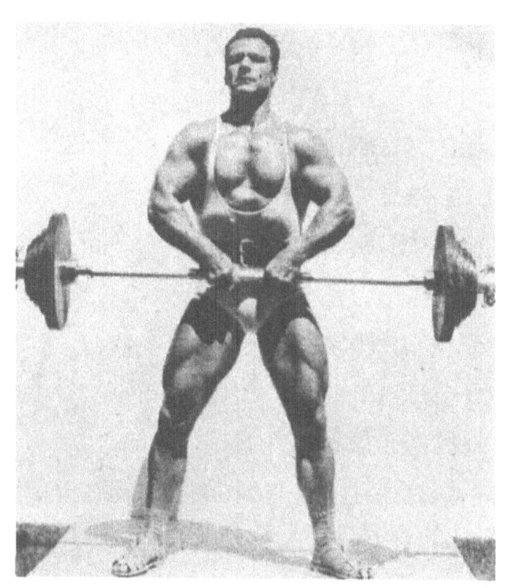 schedules ever invented. The routine itself evolved from the basic weight lifting programs of the York Barbell Club and other lifting schools of the 1930's and 40's that produced Olympic lifter like **John Grimek**, who was successful in both Olympic lifting and Physique Culture (Bodybuilding) at the time.

When the program was adjusted to that of a pure bodybuilding phase of training it produced great results in both muscle mass, strength and physical performance. You were not only strong but you also now looked the part. This was a stark contrast to the old strong men of the past who more than often resembled an barrel with legs and had very little in the way of physical musculature.

Another one of the biggest proponents of the training style was 1947 AAU Mr. America, and 1950 Mr. Universe **Steve Reeves**. Reeves used the 3-day a week program quite extensively during his lifetime as he put it - "This is the best program for adding mass to your physique". Reeves

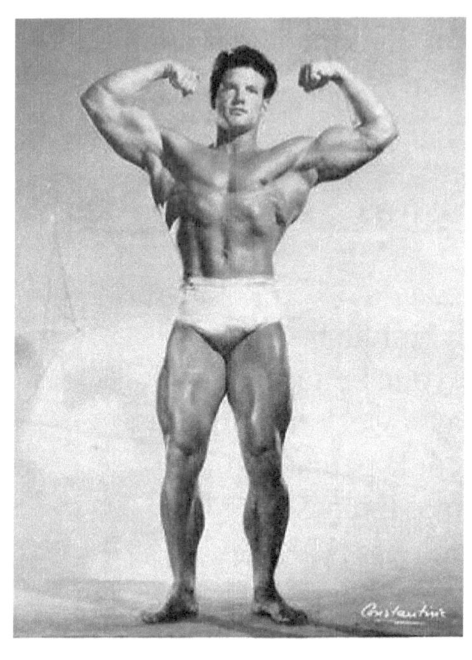

was Arnold S. before there was an Arnold S. He would star in over 15+ movies in his most famous role as legendary strongmen such Hercules, and Sampson through the late 50's up to the late 60's we he would be more into philanthropy. His belief in the 3-day a week training schedule never wavered for a second as it was his training style when he won all his bodybuilding shows and was starring in all those movies. Reeves had the first classic physique the world had ever seen and it was because of this training structure. At a height of 6'1" and a weight of 215 during his competitive days, and 230 pounds after, **Reeves was not a small guy.** He also achieved some pretty sizeable measurement:

- **Height: 6' 1"**
- **Weight: 216**
- **Shoulder Breath: 23 1/2"**
- **Neck: 18 1/2"**
- **Chest: 52"**
- **Waist: 29**
- **Hips: 38"**
- **Biceps: 18 1/4"**
- **Forearms: 14 3/4"**
- **Wrists: 7 1/4"**
- **Thighs: 26"**
- **Calves: 18 1/4"**
- **Ankles: 9 1/4"**

Tell me of any of today physique competitors who would not like to be starting out with these stats. He strived for balance in his physique and in his training. This is why he liked the 3 day overall body approach to training more than any other approach, because it focused on the body as a whole and made you adopt a approach that centered on building a symmetrical and balanced physique.

## <u>Your First Routine</u>

Now that we got you some what attuned to what to wear and basic accessories to bring with you to the gym, we need to set up your training routine and just where we are going to start. We are going to assume that we are starting from scratch with a truly raw recruit. Since you are so new to weight raining the very worst thing for you to do is to adopt one of those routines that are recommended out on social media.

You don't need to worry about counting reps, as all sets will consist of the same rep count except for legs, which will be slightly higher. Your days training will not change for the first **26 weeks** as you will be training your whole body in 3 days, and performing slight stretching and calisthenics the other 2 days with the weekends off to rest and recovery. Your workouts during this phase are designed to stimulate the whole body as it is new to resistance exercise and should adapt to this change quickly during this phase we want to take advantage of this, building your exercise performance, muscular endurance, set recovery.

- **Exercise Performance:** How you execute the exercise and focusing its effects on the target muscles.
- **Muscular Endurance:** Your ability to execute the prescribed number of repetitions, for the required number of sets.
- **Set Recovery:** Your ability to apply full effort to each set of a give exercise beyond the fatigue.

## <u>Basic 3 Day a Week Training Routines:</u>

**Weeks 1-12**

| **Workout #1**: Monday - Emphasis Chest: |
| --- |
| Stationary Bike/Treadmill 5-10 minutes (warm- |

| up) | | |
| --- | --- | --- |
| Exercise | Sets | Reps |
| Bench Press | 3 | 8-12 |
| One DB Arm Row | 3 | 8-12 |
| Upright Rows | 3 | 8-12 |
| Lying French Press | 3 | 8-12 |
| Barbell Curls | 3 | 8-12 |
| Squats | 3 | 8-12 |
| Pullovers | 3 | 8-12 |
| Good Mornings | 3 | 8-12 |

| **Workout #2**: Wednesday - Emphasis Back/Shoulders: | | |
| --- | --- | --- |
| Stationary Bike/Treadmill 5-10 minutes (warm-up) | | |
| Exercise | Sets | Reps |
| Deadlift | 3 | 8-12 |
| One Arm Dumbbell Row | 3 | 8-12 |
| Military Press | 3 | 8-12 |
| Upright Rows | 3 | 8-12 |
| Incline Bench Press | 3 | 8-12 |
| Lying French Press | 3 | 8-12 |
| Barbell Curls | 3 | 8-12 |
| Breathing Squats | 3 | 8-12 |
| Barbell Pullovers | 3 | 8-12 |

| Workout #3: Friday - Emphasis Legs: | | |
| --- | --- | --- |
| Stationary Bike/Treadmill 5-10 minutes (warm-up) | | |
| Exercise | Sets | Reps |
| Squats | 3 | 10-12 |
| Roman Deadlift | 3 | 8-12 |
| Pullovers | 3 | 8-12 |
| Front Pulldown | 3 | 8-12 |
| DB Bench Press | 3 | 8-12 |
| Upright Rows | 3 | 8-12 |
| Triceps Pressdowns | 3 | 8-12 |
| EZ Barbell Curls | 3 | 8-12 |
| Standing Calf Raise | 3 | 12 |

**Workout Notes:** Workouts emphasis should be on getting your workouts completed including all warm-ups with in 45 minutes. You goals should be to add 5- 10 pounds of resistance every 2 weeks while as we have said trying to keep the pace of your training up. These routines are not easy and will challenge even those with workout experience. Concentrate on performing your exercise with complete movements and for the desired number of reps. Use a spotter where needed.

**Active Rest Week** - Week 13: When we say active rest we mean rest with some fitness activities thrown into it such as walking, bike riding, or hiking. These are things that you wouldn't do during a training phase if your trying at acquire muscle mass to any great extent, but are fine during a rest period 2-3 times during the week, with complete rest the last 3 days of the week.

## Weeks 14-25

| Workout #1: Monday - Emphasis Chest: | | |
|---|---|---|
| Stationary Bike/Treadmill 10 minutes (warm-up) | | |
| Exercise | Sets | Reps |
| Bench Press | 3 | 8-12 |
| Incline Bench Press | 3 | 8-12 |
| Bent Barbell Row | 3 | 8-12 |
| Seated Machine Presses | 3 | 8-12 |
| Upright Rows | 3 | 8-12 |
| Lying Extensions | 3 | 8-12 |
| EZ Barbell Curls | 3 | 8-12 |
| Squats | 3 | 8-12 |
| Pull Over | 3 | 8-12 |
| Standing Calf Raises | 3 | 15-20 |

| Workout #2: Emphasis Back/Shoulders: | | |
|---|---|---|
| Stationary Bike/Treadmill 10 minutes (warm-up) | | |
| Exercise | Sets | Reps |
| Dumbbell Swings (warm-up) | 1 | 15-20 |
| Deadlift | 3 | 8-12 |

| Low Pulley Rows | 3 | 8-12 |
| Military Presses | 3 | 8-12 |
| Upright Rows | 3 | 8-12 |
| Incline Bench Press | 3 | 8-12 |
| Breathing Squats | 3 | 20 |
| --- Superset --- | | |
| Barbell Pull Over | 3 | 20 |
| Triceps PressDown | 3 | 10-12 |
| Barbell Curls | 3 | 10-12 |
| Standing Calf Raises | 3 | 15-20 |

| **Workout #3**: Friday - Emphasis Legs: | | |
| --- | --- | --- |
| Stationary Bike/Treadmill 10 minutes (warm-up) | | |
| Exercise | Sets | Reps |
| Barbell Squats | 3 | 8-12 |
| 45Deg Leg Press | 3 | 10-12 |
| Good Mornings | 3 | 8-12 |
| Dumbbell Bench Press | 3 | 8-12 |
| Dumbbell Incline Bench Press | 3 | 8-12 |
| Back Pulldown | 3 | 8-12 |
| Seated DB Presses | 3 | 8-12 |
| Triceps Press Down | 3 | 8-12 |
| Seated Db Curls | 3 | 8-12 |
| Seated Calf Raises | 3 | 15-20 |

**Workout Notes:** As you can see your workouts have changed very slightly from your beginning routine. The emphasis is still on completing your training sessions in a give amount of time. During this phase your time of completion is now 60 minutes. As your workout volume has increased and if you have done a successful job in the first phase so has the amount of weight you are using in each exercise. Mentioning exercises, those to have increased as you are now doing 2 exercise for all the focused muscle groups apposed to the 1 your were doing in the initial phase. This workout phase is the one that separates those who are serious about their training goals and those who just like to dream of getting bigger and stronger. It will be a major challenge to get through your workout in the 60 minutes giving 100% but it can be done and has been done.

**Active Rest Week** - Week 26: When we say active rest we mean rest with some fitness activities thrown into it such as walking, bike riding, or hiking. These are things that you wouldn't do during a training phase if your trying at acquire muscle mass to any great extent, but are fine during a rest period 2-3 times during the week, with complete rest the last 3 days of the week.

## You're Still a Beginner!

Now that you have completed your initial phase of training you're ready to try some of those routines you see in the magazines and get onstage and show off your hard work. Only one problem with this whole scenario is that you're not ready for that you're still a **BEGINNER!**

Completing those **26 weeks** of consistent steady training has begun to lay the foundation the will take you on to any physical competitions you care to enter. But this is about bodybuilding and in the world of bodybuilding you are still a newborn baby. It takes years of consistent steady training and dietary practices (we will discuss this later) to get you on that stage ready to do battle. No we have just begun to get you ready, our next step now is to bring your training into a more focused approach on each body part.

# Chapter 4 Extended Training

## 4-Day a Week Schedule

With all the love and respect we have for the 3-day a week full body-training schedule we know that it cannot be used forever and must be replaced as the individuals become stronger and his/her abilities to recuperate from workout to workout becomes longer. Unlike Olympic lifting, which is, allot more technique driven; bodybuilding requires a more direct link between the movement and the muscles being worked. This makes the 3-day a week approach detrimental to any bodybuilder looking to maximize muscle size and strength in specific muscle groups. Though great for adding overall body size, it does fall a little short when working on weak points. Basically what I am saying is that 3-days a week full body training will add allot of muscle mass to you aver all body, but 4- day a week split training will help you target where that muscle goes allot more.

## Adding Another Day

When I started teach this program over 20 years ago all I had as a reference where the vintage magazine I collected from the late 50', 60's and 70's as a guide to see how the guys training then were able to push past sticking points and move some very heavy weights. You

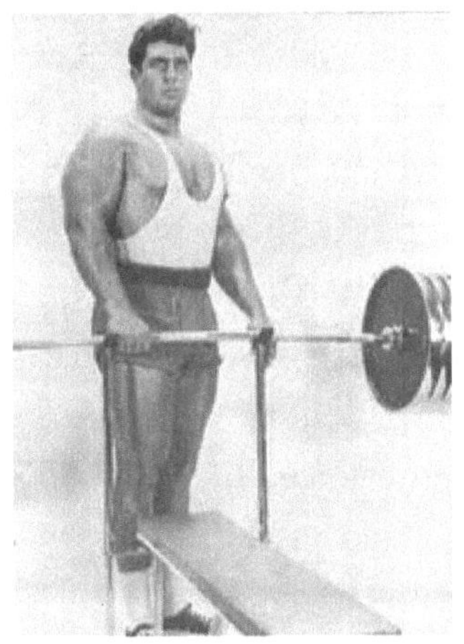

see that most of them were adding sets and doing specialization but the one thing that all those who were achieve greater size and strength gains were doing was adding in more training days with the majority going to 4 days a week training split instead of 3 days a week to get the specialization they wanted. The most successful of them were also splitting body parts and training them 1 or 2 times a week instead of the usual 3 days. The new approach to training was helping bodybuilder and powerlifters of the time reach some lofty heights. Guys were building 20' arms, 60' chest, squatting 750 pounds, and some even benched **600** pounds as the legendary **Pat Casey** did in 1960's. He also became the first man to squat over **800** pounds in a official powerlifting meet. Just think he started out as a bodybuilder from Los Angeles in the 50's.

## **Classic Vs Extended**

This next training phase will see you adding another training day to your workout frequency and splitting up body parts so to more emphasize their growth and recovery to help you add as much muscle mass to your body as you can over the course of each training cycle. You're going to be following a **classic 4-day a week training cycle** that has given some of the greatest bodybuilders of all time their start to stage success.. This is the same type of training schedule used by almost all the greats of the late 50's, 60's and early 70's as it let you keep the 3 day a week approach of yearly years but start to get allot more specific with your body parts. Each body part is trained twice a week instead of 3 full body workouts. With more rest between training sessions, you'll see your strength grow as well as your size. These workouts are the stages where you start o become more of an intermediate bodybuilder than a beginner. Over the course of these next 2 training cycles your body will be seasoned enough for you to start a more specialized training approach geared toward your goals.

**These 4-day a week split routines were the start of all the training concepts you see today** displayed in all the magazine and splashed everywhere on the internet. The **Classic 4-Day Split** which consist of 2 consecutive days with a day off followed by another 2 consecutive day training builds more exercise focus and technique than any routine you can come up with. You have plenty of room to grow and adapt but if learn to concentrate and focus on the working muscle using different exercises on multiple days you will achieve a technique that only a few have conquered. Sorry but you will not develop this with today's micro programmed routines that rely on rep schemes and weight macros to evaluate successful training days. The **Extended 4-Day Split** follows the classic with 2 consecutive training days with a day off but the next 2 training days are split with a rest day in between. Some of the most successful professional bodybuilders of even today use a version of this classic training model. On of the most famous was **6 Time Mr. Olympia Dorian Yates**. The Extended model has the extra edge of a tab bit more rest between second sessions so you can go a little bit heavier and decrease you rep range a little to build more strength and power.

**Classic 4-Day Training Split:**
**Monday** – Chest, Shoulder, Triceps, Abs Calves
**Tuesday** – Legs, Back, Biceps, abs, Calves
**Wednesday** – Rest Day
**Thursday** – Same body parts as Monday different Exercises performed.
**Friday** – Same body parts as Tuesday different Exercises performed.
**Saturday** – Rest Day
**Sunday** – Rest Day

**Extended 4-Day Training Split:**
**Monday** – Chest, Shoulder, Triceps, Abs Calves
**Tuesday** – Legs, Back, Biceps, abs, Calves
**Wednesday** – Rest Day
**Thursday** – Same body parts as Monday different Exercises performed.
**Friday** – Rest Day
**Saturday** – Same body parts as Tuesday different Exercises performed.
**Sunday** – Rest Day

We are going to use both types of training splits over these 2 training cycles starting with the **Classic** split over weeks 27-39 and **Extended** split over weeks 41-52. This will complete our first years training where we will have a 2-week break from all training.

# Classic 4 Day a Week Training Routines:

**Weeks 27-39**

| Workout #1: Monday: Chest, Shoulder Triceps, Calves, Abs | | |
| --- | --- | --- |
| [Warm-up: 10 minutes on exercise bike/treadmill plus light stretching of over all body.] | | |
| Exercise | Sets | Reps |
| Flat Barbell Bench Presses | 4 | 8-15 |
| Incline Barbell Presses | 4 | 8-12 |
| Flat Bench Dumbbell Flyes | 3 | 12-15 |
| Seated Dumbbell Presses | 4 | 8-12 |
| Dumbbell Side Lateral Raises | 3 | 12 |
| Incline Rear Lateral Raises | 3 | 12 |
| Triceps Pressdowns | 3 | 10-12 |
| Dumbbell Triceps Kickbacks | 3 | 12 |
| Standing Calf Raises | 3 | 12-15 |
| Seated Leg Raises | 3 | 15-25 |

| Workout #2: Tuesday: Legs, Back, Biceps, Forearms, Abs | | |
| --- | --- | --- |
| [Warm-up: 10 minutes on exercise bike/treadmill plus light stretching of over all body.] | | |
| Exercise | Sets | Reps |

| 45 Deg. Leg Press | 4 | 12-15 |
|---|---|---|
| Leg Extensions | 3 | 10-12 |
| Lying Leg Curls | 3 | 10-12 |
| T-bar Rows | 4 | 8-12 |
| Front Pulldowns | 3 | 8-12 |
| Hyper Extensions | 3 | 12-15 |
| Standing Barbell Curls | 3 | 8-12 |
| Incline Dumbbell Curls | 3 | 10-12 |
| Barbell Wrist Curls | 3 | 12-15 |
| Roman Chair SitUps | 3 | 12+ |

**Workout #3**: Thursday: Chest, Shoulder Triceps, Calves, Abs

[Warm-up: 10 minutes on exercise bike/treadmill plus light stretching of over all body.]

| Exercise | Sets | Reps |
|---|---|---|
| Incline Dumbbell Presses | 4 | 10-12 |
| Flat Dumbbell Bench Presses | 4 | 10-12 |
| Machine Flyes | 3 | 12-15 |
| Seated Barbell Presses | 3 | 6-12 |
| Wide Grip Upright Rows | 3 | 8-12 |
| Dumbbell Shrugs | 3 | 12 |
| Lying Triceps Extensions | 3 | 10-12 |
| Triceps Dips | 3 | 12-15 |

| Seated Calf Raises | 3 | 12-15 |
|---|---|---|
| Hanging Leg Raises | 3 | 12+ |

| **Workout #4**: Friday: Legs, Back, Biceps, Forearms, Abs | | |
|---|---|---|
| [Warm-up: 10 minutes on exercise bike/treadmill plus light stretching of over all body.] | | |
| Exercise | Sets | Reps |
| Barbell Squats | 4 | 8-12 |
| Dumbbell Lunges | 3 | 12-15 |
| Straight Legged Deadlifts | 3 | 12-15 |
| Chins | 4 | Max Reps BWT |
| Dumbbell Rows | 3 | 10-12 |
| Hyper Extensions | 3 | 12-15 |
| Seated Dumbbell Curls | 3 | 10-12 |
| Barbell Scott Curls | 3 | 10-12 |
| Barbell Reverse Curls | 3 | 12 |
| Standing Cable Crunches | 3 | 15 |

These are classic bodybuilding routines that will produce a maximum response in muscle hypertrophy and at the same time limit the accumulation of excess body fat.

**Workout Notes:** Workouts emphasis should be on getting your workouts completed including all warm-ups with in 60-75 minutes. You goals should always be to add 5- 10 pounds of resistance every 2 weeks while as we have said trying to keep the pace of your training up. These new 4-day routines are not easy and will challenge even those with workout experience. Concentrate on performing your exercise with complete movements and for the desired number of reps listed. These routines give you your first taste of multiple exercises for a single muscle group so concentration that was formed in earlier stages will be very critical here and beyond as workout become more stressful and complicated. Use a spotter where needed.

**Active Rest Week** - Week 40: When we say active rest we mean rest with some fitness activities thrown into it such as walking, bike riding, or hiking. These are things that you wouldn't do during a training phase if your trying at acquire muscle mass to any great extent, but are fine during a rest period 2-3 times during the week, with complete rest the last 3 days of the week.

## Extended 4 Day a Week Training Routines:

**Weeks 41-52**

| Workout #1: Monday: Chest, Shoulder Triceps, Calves, Abs |
| :---: |

| [Warm-up: 10 minutes on exercise bike/treadmill plus light stretching of over all body.] | | |
| --- | --- | --- |
| Exercise | Sets | Reps |
| Flat Dumbbell Bench Presses | 3 | 8-15 |
| Incline Dumbbell Presses | 4 | 8-12 |
| Flat Bench Dumbbell Flyes | 3 | 12-15 |
| Seated Barbell Presses | 4 | 8-12 |
| Dumbbell Side Lateral Raises | 3 | 12 |
| Incline Rear DB Later Raises | 3 | 12 |
| Triceps Pressdowns | 3 | 10-12 |
| Overhead Dumbbell Extensions | 3 | 12 |
| Standing Calf Raises | 3 | 12-15 |
| Seated Leg Raises | 3 | 15-25 |

| **Workout #2**: Tuesday: Legs, Back, Biceps, Forearms, Abs | | |
| --- | --- | --- |
| [Warm-up: 10 minutes on exercise bike/treadmill plus light stretching of over all body.] | | |
| Exercise | Sets | Reps |
| 45 Deg. Leg Press | 4 | 12-15 |
| Leg Extensions | 3 | 10-12 |
| Lying Leg Curls | 3 | 10-12 |
| Deadlifts | 4 | 6-8 |

| Dumbbell Rows | 4 | 8-12 |
|---|---|---|
| Chins | 2 | Max Reps |
| Standing Barbell Curls | 3 | 8-12 |
| Incline Dumbbell Curls | 3 | 10-12 |
| Barbell Wrist Curls | 3 | 12-15 |
| Romain Chair SitUps | 3 | 12+ |

| **Workout #3**: Thursday: Chest, Shoulder Triceps, Calves, Abs | | |
|---|---|---|
| [Warm-up: 10 minutes on exercise bike/treadmill plus light stretching of over all body.] | | |
| Exercise | Sets | Reps |
| Bench Presses | 4 | 6-12 |
| Incline Presses | 4 | 8-12 |
| Machine Flyes | 3 | 12-15 |
| Seated Barbell Presses | 3 | 6-12 |
| Wide Grip Upright Rows | 3 | 8-12 |
| Dumbbell Shrugs | 3 | 12 |
| Lying Triceps Extensions | 3 | 10-12 |
| Triceps Dips | 3 | 12-15 |
| Seated Calf Raises | 3 | 12-15 |
| Hanging Leg Raises | 3 | 12+ |

| **Workout #4**: Saturday: Legs, Back, Biceps, Forearms, Abs | | |
|---|---|---|
| [Warm-up: 10 minutes on exercise bike/treadmill plus light stretching of over all body.] | | |
| Exercise | Sets | Reps |
| Barbell Squats | 5 | 6-10 |
| Leg Extensions | 3 | 10-12 |
| Leg Curls | 3 | 10-12 |
| Chins | 4 | Max Reps BWT |
| Dumbbell Rows | 3 | 10-12 |
| Hyper Extensions | 3 | 12-15 |
| Seated Dumbbell Curls | 3 | 10-12 |
| Barbell Scott Curls | 3 | 10-12 |
| Barbell Reverse Curls | 3 | 12 |
| Standing Cable Crunches | 3 | 15 |

These **4-day extended bodybuilding** routines are designed to not only produce a maximum response in muscle hypertrophy but also advance your strength curve with the use of lower rep ranges on multi-joint exercise to recruit a different kind of muscle fiber to farther stimulate growth. This stage of training also provides a bridge toward the Phase Training techniques you will be using through out your next year of training and beyond. Extended training also just like classic helps you limit the accumulation of excess body fat.

**Workout Notes:** Workouts emphasis should be on getting your workouts completed including all warm-ups with in 60-75 minutes. You goals should always be to add 5- 10 pounds of resistance every 2 weeks while as we have said trying to keep the pace of your training up. These new 4-day routines are not easy and will challenge even those with workout experience. Concentrate on performing your exercise with complete movements and for the desired number of reps listed. These routines give you your first taste of multiple exercises for a single muscle group so concentration that was formed in earlier stages will be very critical here and beyond as workout become more stressful and complicated. Use a spotter where needed.

**Active Rest Week** - Week 40: When we say active rest we mean rest with some fitness activities thrown into it such as walking, bike riding, or hiking. These are things that you wouldn't do during a training phase if your trying at acquire muscle mass to any great extent, but are fine during a rest period 2-3 times during the week, with complete rest the last 3 days of the week.

# Chapter 5 Phased Training

Now that you have your first years under your belt you are now what we old timers call a intermediate bodybuilder. You are more than a beginner, but less than an advanced trainer. You are in the sweet spot as now we get to experiment with all kinds of techniques to enhance your training, and **NO** we are not talking about pharmaceuticals (Drugs). We are talking about training techniques, kind of training cycles, cycle duration, Targeted workouts to shape your physique, workouts to restructure your physique. Being a teenage bodybuilder is very unique opportunity that if directed in positive directions can lead to great things down the line. As they say in my generation lets get Crackin.

## Cycled Training

When we talk about cycled training we're talking about putting your training on a different mission during each training period. Each of these periods are usually broken down into 12 weeks long as that is the kind of generalized time frame it usually take for the body to workup to a peak and gradually plateau before needing a rest to recovery from the stress of the training. This is the main reason when you started this program your training was and is based on 12-week periods with active rest in between. You're putting the body on this wave of progression that it will only see once because you are so new and fresh to resistance training. This period is doubly important that you take full advantages of your earliest stages so they pay big dividends later.

Progress is never a straight line progression from point A to point B. Have you noticed that when you come back from a good rest you're actually starting out below where you left off. Don't try to push it to hard because this is a normal process and should be expected. It usually takes about 5.5 weeks for your body to fully be back into a grove that feels familiar. This is called your inflection point of the cycle. It's the actual time where you start to see progress over the last training cycle or Supercompesation. This will usually peak around week 8 or 9, with weeks 10 and beyond regressing slightly but also solidifying progress. Unlike what you hear or see on the Internet none of that micro manage so-called programs are going to keep you from tapering off at the end of a training cycle. It doesn't and NEVER has worked like that.

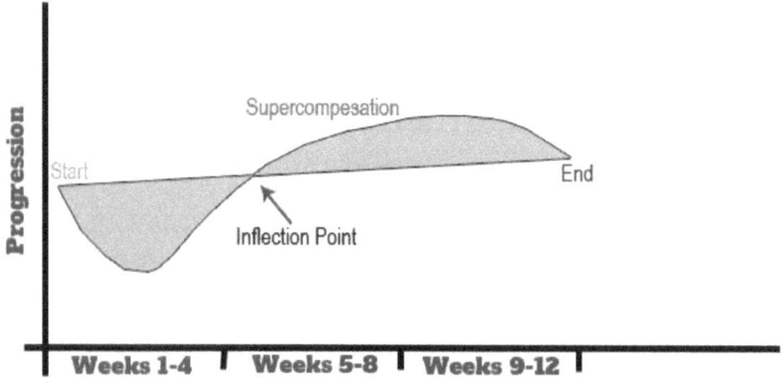


During this years training we are going to do allot of great things. Build limit strength and power, get cut up and contest ready, plus maximize hypertrophy with targeted routines and intensity techniques, all to help us put some finishing touches on our training subconscious so we have the platform to step into advanced levels of training and continue to progress and not stagnate and fail as more than 90% do. That's a high number, but it is an accurate number because talent only goes so far, it's what you have done and what you know that get you into that upper percentile. Easier said, you got to put in the WORK!

## Reshaping Your Body

Now lets be clear when we talk about re-shaping your body we're not talking about stretching you out another 2-3 inches in height, or shortenings your legs or lengthening your torso. When we talk about changing the shape of your body we mean using exercise to help you maximize areas in your physique to help you grow those areas to provide a look the better reflect the ideal structure. As a young bodybuilder your body is not yet set in stone so we can to some extent help you increase or decrease certain areas with targeted exercise grouping to do just that.

Being that most person under the age of 23 are still growing to some extent it would be of interest to them to be able to focus on certain areas to help build a structure that is more closely related to the ideal standard of bodybuilding. We have put in our top 4 specific routines that can be plug into your training routine for one of the body parts workout of the week to help enhance your overall shape.

## <u>Body Part Re-Shaping Routines:</u>

**Stretching and Expanding The Ribcage:** This is a super-set exercise combination that involves Barbell Squats & Straight Bar Pullovers. Now most people believe they know how to do this but the efforts I have seen in most gyms and training session fall way short. We are going to explain just how to do this to get the most benefit from the combination, when done right it is very effective over the course of 6 months to expand the rib box about 3-5 inches. That creates a dramatic change in chest size and shape.

**Set Up:**
*Equipment* - Load the squat bar with a weight which you can complete 20 reps with in normal fashion with not much effort. Next to the squat rack place a flat bench and a barbell of very light (just enough to where you can feel it: about 20Lbs). You will needs these to be close to each other as you will be moving between exercise with little to no rest until all sets are performed.

*Squats* - Place two 5-pound plates on the floor about shoulder width apart, these will be full squats all the way down and all the way up. The plates under your heals

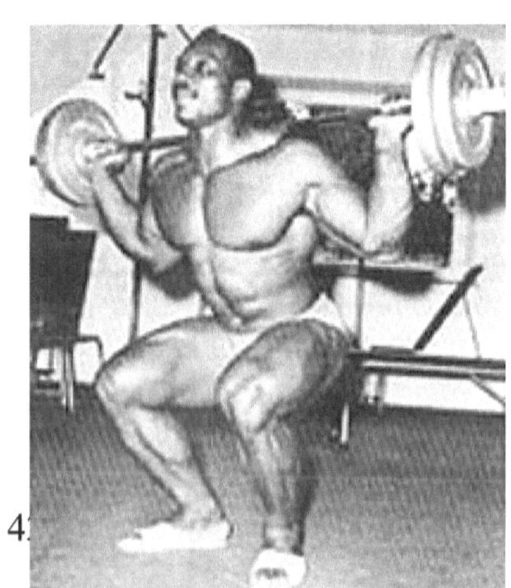

place more of the emphasis onto the front of the thighs and reduces strain on the hips. Use a weight that is 50% of your heaviest workout weight. In the start position squat all the way down to the bottom and return to the starting position and take 2 deep breathes, then squat again. Repeat this for 20 reps, taking 2 deep breathes between each rep. At around rep 15 your breathing will start getting heavier but focus and complete all 20 reps in the same fashion. Move on directly to Straight Arm Barbell Pullovers.

*Barbell Pullovers* - Lying length wise on a flat bench with your arms extended straight up grasp a light barbell with your hands about shoulder width apart, keep your back flat on the bench (Don't arch as this decreases the stretch) take a deep breathe and hold it as your lower the bar in a circular arc keeping your arms as straight as possible until it is level with your torso and return to the top exhaling along the way. Take 2 deep breathes and repeat the exercise for 20 reps. Move directly back to Squats with as little rest as possible continue until 3 super-sets are done with as little rest as possible between sets.

Workout Tips: This routine is not about using heavy weights or trying to impress anyone. This routine is about creating a larger chest cavity by placing stress both internal and external on the ribcage through heavy breathing and progressive stretching. Follow this routine for 6 weeks before switching back to regular workouts.

**Widening and Developing the Chest:** Having a full ribcage is very impressive but your going to need to cover that with thick slabs of muscle from top to bottom and from side to sternum. To do this we are going to rely on 2 exercises again that most will feel that they know how to perform but not in the way we do to maximize muscle growth over just satisfying your ego. The first exercise will be Wide Grip Bench Presses, immediately followed be Chest Dips. The combination when done right will add width and thickness to your pecs from all angles to give you that complete developmental look of a champion competitive bodybuilder.

**Set Up:**

*Equipment* - Load the bench press with a weight that you can use for 12 reps in normal fashion with not to much effort. Locate the dipping bars and place a towel on them if it's a walk away to let others know you're going to be using the equipment. Do not use a machine for your dips, as these are not the same exercise. You want the free movement of the bars as this recruits more muscle fiber and provides a better stretch and contraction.

*Wide Grip Bench Press* - Adjust yourself onto the bench press, as you would do normally. Now we want you to slide back about a inch farther, this helps with not placing to much stress on the shoulder when un-racking the weight with a slightly wider grip. Now grip the bar as you would normally, moves your hands out 2 inches on each side. This put your grip into a wide grip placement. Do 2 warm-up sets with this grip before 3 working set that will be super-set with parallel bar Chest Dips to be described next. Keep the weight in the medium range, as we want to build muscle mass and not set powerlifting records. We do want you to use enough weight though to limit you reps to a maximum of 12, as this will become harder on succeeding sets. Perform 10-12 reps with a 1 second pause and squeeze at the top of the movement on each repetition. Up on completion of your set of 12 reps you go as quickly as you can to Chest Dip where you complete as many as possible with only bodyweight.

*Chest Dips -* When performing Chest Dips we want to place the emphasis of the movement onto the chest and away from the triceps and limit the shoulder as 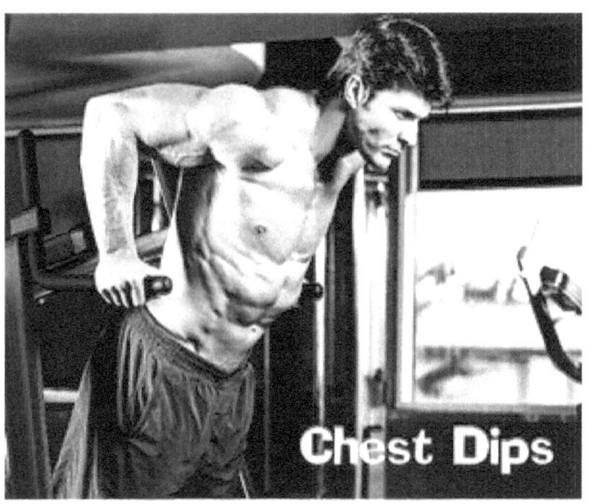

much as possible. At the top of the movement with your arms straight tuck your head until your chin touches your chest. This will cause your body to tilt slightly forward, which is exactly what we want. Now with your arm straight descent downward by lower yourself chest first until your upper arms are parallel with the floor feeling the stretch in your lower and outer chest, now push back up forcefully contracting your chest first and a slight bit of triceps to the starting position. You should feel these in your chest from start to finish because of the forward lean created from tucking your chin to chest (Keep Your Chin Tucked). Perform as many reps as possible with bodyweight. Return to the bench press to ready your self for the next set.

Oh Yeah you get to rest for 3 second between super sets here as the auxiliary muscles here aren't as strong as your legs in the previous grouping. Repeat for 3 super sets with 30 seconds rest in between. Use this combination at the beginning of your chest workout and augment with 1 or 2 other shaping exercises to finish the chest workout. Follow this routine for 6 weeks before switching back to regular workouts.

**Widening and Developing the Shoulders and Traps:** Having wide shoulder with big side deltoids and thick sweeping traps is one of the hallmarks of a successful bodybuilder. Getting those attributes is harder for many people that are not born with the ideal bone structure of say a Dorian Yates or Ronnie Coleman. Even with these shortcomings we can add length to the width to your shoulders, plus thicken your trap. With the use of Wide Grip Chins and Dumbbell Shrugs you can give yourself the broad shoulders and V-taper that help to make for a championship physique.

**Set Up:**
*Equipment* - Your going to need a pair of wrist straps for these. For this set of exercises you're going to need them because your grip will fail you before the

target muscles. Grab yourself a flat bench and place it next to the Chinning bar. On the bench you're going to place 2 dumbbells of medium heavy weight for use on your shrugs. We use the bench to keep you from having to bend over during the super set and help preserve your lower back muscles.

*Wide Grip Chins* - When performing a wide grip chin to affect your shoulder your going to go really wide, we're talking about 6-8 inches beyond shoulder width. Using a stool or the edge of the bench position yourself and get strapped in tight before stepping off the bench hang for a second count to bend your knees back and cross your feet. Pull yourself up as high as you can, clear at least your chins above the bar. Return to the bottom and allow for a 1-2 second stretch before perfuming another rep. If you can not clear your chin use assistance to go as high as possible and complete 10 reps. Drop down and immediately move over to the Dumbbell Shrugs.

*Dumbbell Shrugs* - Move over to the dumbbells and quickly strap up lifting them to your side with palms facing your thighs. Tilt your torso very slightly forward feeling the strain of the weight across the back of the shoulders. Pull your shoulders up as high as possible using just your trapezius muscles, squeezing at the top before returning to the bottom stretch. Perform 10 reps in controlled fashion with traps as the prime movers.

You're going to perform 3 super sets 10 reps with each movement. Allow yourself 30-second rest between super sets. This is a great super set for widen your shoulders and building the traps at the same time. Follow this routine for 6 weeks before switching back to regular workouts.

**Building Big Arms:** If there was one thing every Teenage or Young Bodybuilder has in his or her mind is building up their arms. Guys may want to build their to crazy sizes, but girls also want to build theirs arms just as much only not so big. The tried and true exercises to help you build your arms up are Lying Triceps Extension & Power Curls with a Straight Bar.

Set Up:
Equipment - 2 Barbells loaded with weights that allow for 8-10 reps. You will also need a flat exercise bench for the triceps extensions.

*Lying Triceps Extension* - With a straight bar we are going to take a grip that's about 6-8 inches apart. Place it on your legs as you sit down on the flat bench. In one motion as you begin to lay back on the bench kip the barbell up to arms length over your torso. With your elbows locked in a 90 deg angle slowly lower the bar toward your forehead in semi-circle fashion until its about an inch from touching your head began to press it back up using your triceps along the same arc. Perform 8 reps and go straight into Power Curls.

*Power Curls* - Now Power Curls are just like regular barbell curls but we going to extent the set by cheating a little to get those extra reps we want with the heavier weight. The barbell should be loaded with weight that limits the amount of strict reps to about 5-6. Up on reaching your limit you are going to use a little nudge from your lower back and legs to get the weight moving to the top of the movement. At the top your going the resist the weight going down for a 3-4 second negative or return to the starting position before cheating again for 2 more reps in similar fashion. That's a total of 5-6 strict reps along with 3 cheat reps.

You're going to perform 3 super set with each movement. Allow yourself 30-second rest between super sets. This is a time proven super set for thickening your arms. Follow this routine for 4-6 weeks before switching back to regular workouts.

## Super Sets, Drop Sets & Forced Reps

As you have read in the previous sections we have inserted the use or super-sets to help increase the intensity of the workout to produce more muscle growth. Super Sets along with Drop Sets and Forced Reps are the most effective form of Intensity Modifiers that work at any level of training. These are the best of the best intensity techniques to help your achieve extra growth, increased muscular endurance, and explosive muscle power. These methods, though they may be old, work better than many so called modern intensity increaser, which are almost always somewhat based on one of them.

**Intensity Modifiers:**

*Super Sets:* This involves 2 different exercise done back-to-back with as little amount of rest between exercise. Usually the 2 muscle groups are antagonist to each other to stretch one as the other contracts. One of the most common super set body parts is 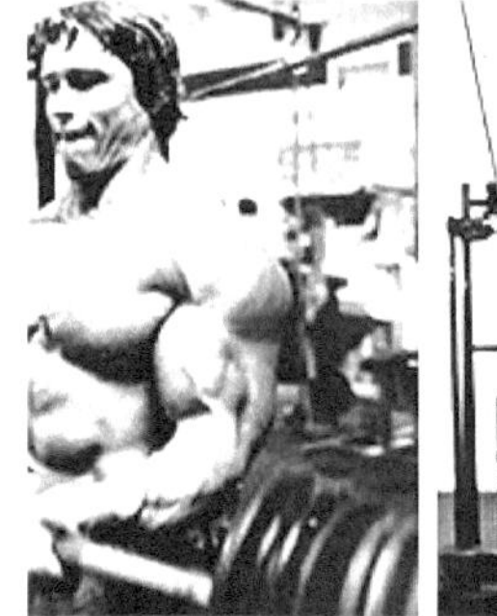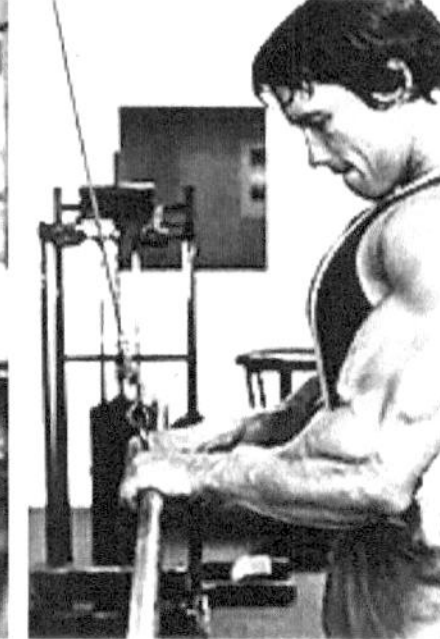 biceps and triceps, because it provides a fuller and more complete pump in your arms. Super set can involve exercise that both target the same muscle groups but from different angles like barbell curls super-set with Incline curls or bench presses super-set with flat dumbbell flyes. The key is that it 2 exercises performed back to back with little rest between them.

*Drop Sets:* Drop sets are one of the best ways to target stubborn muscles that don't respond to just doing regular sets and reps. Drop sets involve you doing your first part of the set as usual. You perform say 10 reps on the bench press failing on the 10th rep. Instead of getting off the bench and setting up for your next set you quickly move to lower the weight and proceed to perform more repetitions again til failure, again stripping a little more weight and doing another set til failure. This is a drop set done with a weighted barbell. Drop sets provide overload on all the working muscles of the target exercise. These are great for stubborn muscle groups like Calves,

Forearms, Upper Back, and Deltoid muscles. These are muscle that recovery quickly and can take the trauma delivered from the technique. This is not to say that doing drop sets on other groups cannot be beneficial, as they to may need a jump-start from time to time.

*Forced Repetitions:* Forced Repetitions are probably one of the most over used and wrongly use intensity techniques in use today. Lets first talk about what a forced rep set is and what it is not. Forced reps are done at the very end of your regular set. When you hit muscular failure and can't perform another complete repetition under your own power, you receive just enough assistance from your training partner to complete another repetition. The amount of force applied is just enough to help you complete between 2-3 extra reps. Forced repetitions should only be performed on your last set of an exercise set. If you do 4 sets of bench presses forced reps are performed on the 4th set. What forced reps are not is something that is used on every set of an exercise. Forced reps are not applicable on every exercise. They work great on multi-joint exercises like bench presses, squats and Standing Barbell Curls. *They can be done but are not great for smaller muscle groups, or isolation exercise* **Scott Curls** *or* **Dumbbell Flyes** *where injuries are more adapt to occur.*

## **Balancing Your Physique**

One of the most common problems beginner and novice body builder get into is training body parts they like harder than those that don't respond as easy with the same intensity. This is the fastest way to lead to an unbalanced physique. We have all seen them, the guy with a good-sized upper body and legs that look like match sticks. You will never achieve your bodybuilding goals preferring one body part to another. This

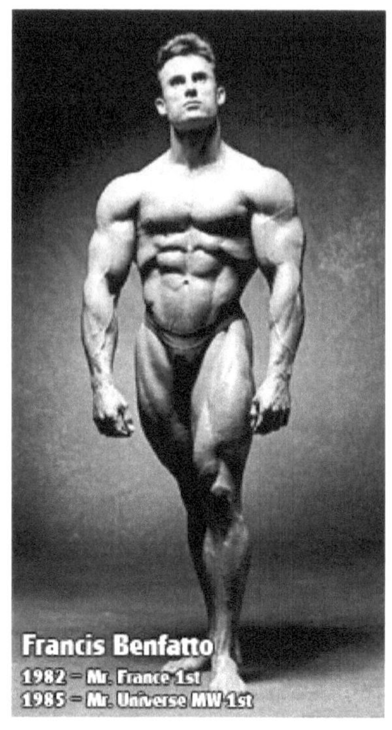



is where you get to use those **Intensity modifiers** mentioned earlier. These help you get stubborn body parts moving in the right direction. Always strive for balance to create a physique that looks many times bigger than it always is, this is the illusion of bodybuilding. Some people use a percentage of certain measurements to predicate how big a body part should be. Steve Reeves used this method to sculpt his physique. We prefer to have different body parts be similar in size to other which balances your look no matter bodyweight or height. We provide both methods for your use. Using the balance charts below to help keep you body parts from getting to big or help bring up other lagging behind.

## Steeve Reeves Muscle to Joint Measurement Muscle To Measurement Ratios:

- Arm size = 252% of wrist size
- Calf size = 192% of ankle size
- Neck Size = 79% of head size
- Chest Size = 148% of hips size
- Waist size = 86% of hips size
- Thigh size = 175% of knee size

## MuscleSports Body Part to Body Part Balancing Chart

- Arm Size - Neck Size - Calf Size: All measure with .5 inches of each other.
- Thigh is 1.5 time the size of you Calf
- Chest is 1.6 times the size of your Waist

**All these measurements are in contest ready conditioning**

## Your 4 Key areas to watch:

- ❑ Calves
- ❑ Forearms
- ❑ Neck
- ❑ Waist

Keeping your eyes on these 4 areas will help you greatly in making sure your physique stays balanced and competition ready.

# Chapter 6 Nutrition Concepts

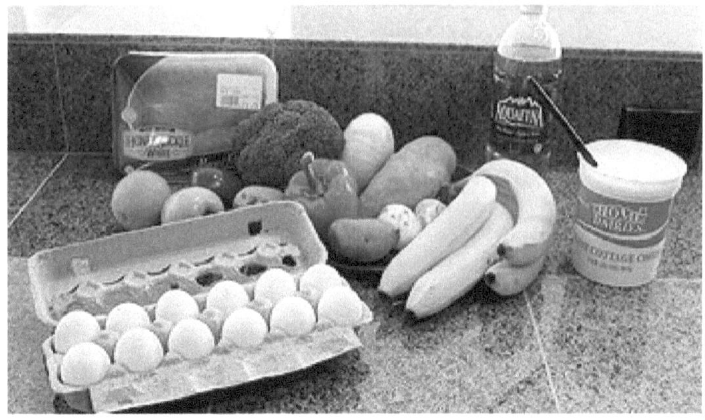

As a teenage or very young bodybuilder one of the most demanding things for youngsters to grasp is the concept of how important nutrition really is to their improvement and growth as an athlete and a bodybuilder. Even more than training, nutrition is the most important part of your bodybuilding life. Being young bodybuilders you are dealing with things older bodybuilders aren't dealing with, school (high school or college), going places with friends and having a social life outside of training. On top of that every single fast food advertisement is targeted directly at you. Getting your nutritional concepts on solid footing is of the utmost importance to achieving the goals you have set for your self as a bodybuilding athlete. Follow these concepts will help you be able to have a more healthy nutritional eating plan, plus it lets you have a active social life.

# Basic Nutrition Rules

We know everyone has an app for all thing nutrition so answer this question for us here at MuscelSports.net: If everyone and their brother knows so damn much about nutrition than why is this world so **F@CKING FAT**! The answer is that even with all the technology in the world 98% of everyone on this planet doesn't have a clue as to what rules govern having a clean and healthy nutritional eating plan. For all those in the Bedrock Bodybuilding program you will know the basic rules of clean and constructive eating for muscle growth and fat loss. Follow these rules during your everyday activities and plan all meals accordingly and you should be able to keep your progress on the correct path.

*DRINK PLENTY OF WATER!* We know that you hear this allot, but for a bodybuilder or any training athlete drinking plenty of water everyday is very important. Water of course helps remove toxins from the body, but it also hydrates the muscles and helps with nutrient adsorption. Hard training bodybuilders should get at least 1- 1½ gallon a day. Yeah I know we said gallon, so keep track of your water intake and make sure you stay well hydrated.

*No samples.* Ever go to say **Costco** or **Sams Club** and see the demo people and you say I'll just sample a little. You don't sample a little, you come around two three time until you pretty much had a whole piece of what being demoded. Or are you just say to your self I'll just have a little piece and before you know it the whole cookie, slice of cake, or tub of ice cream is gone. Stay away form tasting food that you're not supposed to have. Block it out of your mind.

*Remove all excess sugar from your diet.* We don't mean cut all carbohydrates from your diet but remove those extras that you don't need. You know the ones the sodas, fruit juices, and all simple sugar condiments. You know where all those extra sugars go don't you? There not building any mass, oh no there being stored as good old fat. Try drinking water or milk instead.

*Keep your starchy carbs to a minimum.* Removing processed carbs such as breads, cereals, and grains from your diet will help with excess fat being stored on the body. Keep your carb meals early in the day when energy is need for work and exercise. Decrease them as the day progress and try not to eat any right before bedtime. This will help you remove belly fat and those pesky love handles; we know you want those gone.

*Make your last meal a protein one.* One good way to do this is to have a protein shake before going to bed. A good protein shake with casein protein will take time to digest and is a excellent way to nourish your muscles as you sleep. Another trick we find that works if all you have is whey protein
is to add at least 1 tablespoon of peanut butter to your shake. The fat will slow the digestion of the protein

and help spread nutrients over a longer period of time.

*Remove saturated fats from your diet.* Saturated fatty acids are those that are usually hard at room temperature. Saturated fatty acids are very hard for the human body to digest and usually end up stored as fat because of this. Things that have a lot of saturated fat are cheese, 2% to whole milk, and pretty much all processed meats. You still need essential fatty acids, these can be found in eggs, fish, and nuts.

*Eat at least five or six meals throughout the day.* This will keep your body's metabolism burning at a high rate. This also will allow you to vary protein choices and to adjust caloric intake depending on the time of day. Eating just 3 meals a day makes each meal quite large and is not good for your metabolism. Enough said.

*Meal Timing.* Eat at least one carb meal and one protein meal before your workouts. Most important meal is right after your workout. After your workout drink a quality protein shake and have another carb meal, maybe a bowl of oatmeal with some honey about a tablespoon with a banana or strawberries. This provides your body with the needed nutrients at the right time.

*Do cardio on your days off.* Doing cardio on your days off keeps you metabolism churning at a high pace allowing for more calories to be burn. Try limiting your session to 20-30 minutes.

*Take a multi-vitamin and If you can swing it, take L-Glutamine.* This will help prevent muscle loss while on a restrictive eating plan. Eating for bodybuilding is a restrictive eating plan. Apply these rules, and you will be shedding pounds of unwanted body fat and gaining muscle.

Theses rules are not made to be easy so yeah it's going to be tough. We said at the beginning of the chapter that nutrition is the hardest thing for everyone to conquer in their bodybuilding journey and these very basic rules are part of the reason why, they are all well away from the norm of society. If you want to be more than the normal person and being a champion bodybuilder is quite far from the norm than you must master these rules and the discipline they require in your daily life.

## <u>All Proteins are not the Same</u>

Protein is the single most important nutrient to a aspiring young bodybuilder. You can afford to have a deficiency of all other nutrient categories for a certain period of time and still not fell its ill effects, but with protein its like a car with no wheels, you aren't going nowhere. Proteins make and maintain most of the stuff in our bodies. Proteins are differently arranged strands cells called amino acids. They serve as the major structural component of your muscles and other tissues in the body. In addition, amino acids are used to produce hormones, enzymes and hemoglobin in the blood. Your body can also convert protein to energy when all other sources have been depleted. This is a very catabolic state where you are literally living off your own muscle tissue to survive. As a bodybuilder this is the extreme opposite of what you want. So believe ***PROTEIN IS VERY IMPORTANT TO YOUR PROGRESS***.

Here at MuscleSports.net you know that we don't believe in bullshit supplements and over stuffing you with "how you need this and that to be successful". Certain supplements (which we will talk about in a future book) are needed at certain times. With protein you will never hear us say you need to take in more than 0.8 to 1.2 grams per pound of the stuff a day, with the higher end being for elite level competitors and not the average trainer. We are not going to be recommending any 400 or 500 grams of the stuff a day because that shit is just crazy. Over consumption like that leads to bloating and all sorts of gastric and kidney problems you don't won't, trust us. With that out of the way lets get started.

For proteins to be used by the body they need to be metabolized into their simplest form, amino acids. There have been 20 amino acids identified that are needed for human growth and metabolism. Twelve of these amino acids (eleven in children) are termed nonessential, meaning that they can be synthesized by our body and do not need to be consumed in the diet. The remaining amino acids cannot be synthesized in the body and are described as essential meaning that they need to be consumed in our diets. The absence of any of these amino acids will compromise the ability of tissue to grow, be repaired or be maintained.[1]

Don't let anyone tell you that protein isn't the most important nutrient in your training nutritional program. Using the guide above as your reference point, a 200lb off-season bodybuilder would need to intake 240 grams of protein a day at the highest. Protein should make up 35% of your daily intake with carbs at 45% and high quality fats rounding everything out at 20%. This nutrient markup is ideal for the cultivation of muscular mass. A typical daily caloric intake of a 200lb bodybuilder in the off-season, it would be broken down as follows:

240g of Protein - 4 calories per gram of Protein

308g of Carbohydrates - 4 calories per gram of Carbohydrates

61g of Fat - 9 calories per gram of Fat

-------------------------------------------------

= 2742 Calories

Now that you have a good idea of how much protein to consume on a daily basis lets look at the many different kinds of protein source the you have to choose from and what their Protein Efficiency Ratio is when compared to others. Now most articles your have probably read talks about Biological Value which is good but we want to know how good is the protein when you eat it, not how good it stacks up when looking at the structure in chemical terms. The chart below shows you the most popular protein choice among athletes and how they score on usage with in your body.

Protein Quality Rankings.

| Protein Type | Protein Efficiency Ratio | Biological Value | Net Protein Utilization | Protein Digestibility Corrected Amino Acid Score |
|---|---|---|---|---|
| Beef | 2.9 | 80 | 73 | 0.92 |
| Black Beans | 0 | | 0 | 0.75 |
| Casein | 2.5 | 77 | 76 | 1.00 |
| Egg | 3.9 | 100 | 94 | 1.00 |
| Milk | 2.5 | 91 | 82 | 1.00 |
| Peanuts | 1.8 | | | 0.52 |
| Soy protein | 2.2 | 74 | 61 | 1.00 |
| Wheat gluten | 0.8 | 64 | 67 | 0.25 |
| Whey protein | 3.2 | 104 | 92 | 1.00 |

Adapted from: U.S Dairy Export Council, Reference Manual for U.S. Whey Products 2nd Edition, 1999 and Sarwar, 1997.

Looking at the above chart would indicate that the use of Whey Protein would be the very best way for you to go in your pursuit of providing your self with the best protein source for muscle growth. As with all scientific charts the human body does not work like analysis in a petrie dish. Whey protein, though a good additive to your eating plan should never be the main source of the protein you consume during your day. Your goals for daily protein intake should be centered on animal, dairy and vegetable protein sources. These sources provide many macro and micronutrients along with the amino acid profile you need to build muscle mass at a much high rate than depending on just Whey to do the whole job. Below is a listing of the food protein choices from which your should be centering your nutritional plan around:

**Best Protein Choices:**
Beef, Chicken Breast, Chicken Thighs, Turkey Breast, Turkey Drumsticks, Eggs (Whole, Whites), Milk (Whole, Raw), Fish (Salmon, Cod, Trout, Tuna, Sardines, & Mackerel), Cottage Cheese, and Old Fashion Yogurt Plain (Greek Yogurt)

All of these choices provide your physique with more than just protein. If you need to substitute for a meal because of time crunch problems and can't sit down for a meal, then you add in a whey protein shake. Now lets talk about workout energy.

## Fueling your Workouts

When we talk about fueling your workouts we are not talking about the new fangled pre-workout supplement that has hit the market just this week. We are talking about real fuel for your workouts that drive you through some of the heaviest training sessions that you may have, during some of the harshest time of the year. Do you think some caffeine loaded pre-workout crap is going to get you through a set of

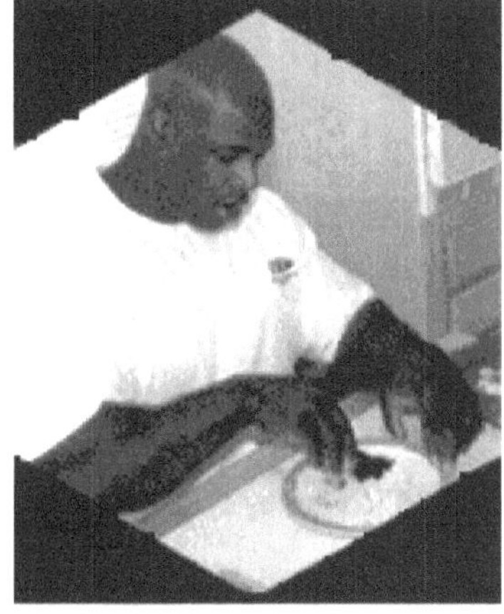

maximum squats during the dog days of summer? That shit will leave you having spasms in a corner somewhere because the extreme heat combined with the high dosed of caffeine has your head about to explode. When we here at MuscleSports.net talk workout fuel we are talking about carbohydrates. Preferably we are talking complex carbohydrates to be exact. Carbs get you through your workouts, and help jump-start the growth process after your workouts. Protein and amino acids are the building blocks of muscle and carbohydrates are the cement that holds the walls together (along with good fats).

Let's get something straight, when we are talking about carbohydrates we are not talking about the refined carb crap that everyone likes to stuff their fat face with such as: ice cream, sweet cereals, pasta, bread, cakes and candy. These carbs are filled with refined sugar that your body does not utilize efficiently or effectively and cause massive health problems. These carbs are the ultimate in failure to your bodybuilding goals. They will make you fat and deliver NOTHING to you!

When we talk about carbs we are talking about low glycemic carbs such as oatmeal, sweet potatoes, yams, brown rice, and high glycemic carbs like, white potatoes, dextrose, maltodextrin, grits, and cream of rice. Fibrous carbs such as broccoli, cauliflower, string beans, asparagus, and mushrooms also serve a purpose to keep your energy level up and to aid in digestion. Along with leafy greens that provide phytonutrients, minerals and an array of vitamins like kale, spinach, collards, cabbage, beets, celery, onions, and many more leafy vegetables. Every one of these sources provides essential benefits to your daily bodybuilding nutrition.

Allot of people are very unfamiliar with the best times to consume carbohydrates to get the most from them towards your workouts. The very best time is in the early morning with your first meal. Usually having a low glycemic carb such as oatmeal (Yeah we know it sounds boring, but it works) will keep your energy levels up through the day, and does not spike your insulin levels making you feel all drowsy. Eating a low glycemic carb like oatmeal will actually help in the body keeping you awake throughout the early parts of the day. In addition, lower glycemic carbs burn more efficiently and keep your muscle fuller longer during workout, and recovery. Sweet potatoes are a good choice of a carb for your second and third meals of the day; this is assuming that you are eating on time every three hours. Your third food meal should be at least 4 hours before your workout so as to clear all foods out of the gut before training.

The meal your going to have pre-training will probably be a liquid meal in the form of a protein/carbohydrate shake. It should be consumed at least 1 to 1.5 hour before training. Even though a liquid meals such as this does pass through the gut quicker than regular food we still don't want anything that resembles some of the stimulant driven so call pre-workout stuff you see on the market today. These drinks are out for only one thing - **YOUR MONEY!** Below is one of the best pre-workout drinks you'll every have. It provides both energy and the nutrients to fuel your muscles from the beginning to the end of your workouts.

**Pre-Workout Drink:**
- 30 Grams Whey Isolate Protein (Chocolate/Vanilla)
- 10 Grams Dextrose
- 5 Grams L-Citrulline
- 3 Grams Creatine Monohydrate

**Consume 1 to 1.5 hours before training – Mix with 12oz of water.**

Finial note - if carbs are utilized properly and strategically placed in your diet, they will add energy, keep you strong throughout your workouts. Your muscles will look full pumped and strong during and after your training. A lack of good carbs in your diet is why you see allot of those guys running around drinking these so called energy/pre-workout drinks looking like strung out beanpoles. Utilizing your carbs like this will keep you lean, and full energy levels through the roof. Fibrous carbs should be utilized throughout the day to aid in digestion of all the protein that you are consuming.

**Yeah**, protein is important when it comes to building and maintaining muscle. But carbohydrates are just as important because they fuel your body and aid in recovery post workout. Whether you are in the off-season or twelve weeks out from a show, carbohydrates need to be utilized in order to achieve your goals. After all, you don't bust your ass everyday for nothing.

## Structured Meals

**Structured Meals** is the practice of planning out your daily nutritional intake into a structured plan that has you feeding your body at certain time of the day to ensure the feeding of your body as far as basic needs is met on a daily basis. This is the clinical explanation for structured eating. Most of you probably didn't know that the concept has been around for about 70-80 years as it was first introduced to make sure persons with eating disorders ingested enough nutrients daily to not harm themselves. You see it used to treat Anorexia, Bulimia and other disorders. For our purposes as bodybuilders we use this to insure that we don't have nutrient deficiencies not for the lack of food but for the growth of muscle mass and recovery due to weight training and aerobic activity.

**The basic components of Structured Meals are these:**

- ❑ **When to eat:** Eating of a meal every 3 hours of the day. 5 meals at least eaten every day
- ❑ **What to eat at each meal:** A consistent amount of Protein, Carbohydrates, and Fats from as clean and natural of food sources as possible with little to no processing.
- ❑ **How much to consume at each meal:** Total caloric macro breakdown of nutrient total for each meals, each day, and each week.

When to eat: All bodybuilder have learned the rule of thumb of eating every 3 hours to keep the body anabolic, its been printed in just about every mag article you have seen for the last 20 years. Most believed it came from some mythical guru who just sat down and figured it out, but it did not it came from the study of diabetics and normalizing their blood sugar levels. Research found that those who ate every 3-4 hour interval had a more normalized blood sugar level and reduced insulin level spikes. Eating more frequent as discussed by allot of the Guru's of the day will only result in wasted consumption, a bloated gut, and excess stored body fat do to insulin spikes (which are exactly what you don't want from your meals). Eating within the first hour of waking is a very good rule of thumb to practice, this breaks the fasting from sleep and allows your body to move into more anabolic state and increases metabolism. Below is a sample-feeding schedule you can use to help space out your meals throughout the day:

Wake @ 6:30 AM
Meal #1 - 7:30 AM
Meal #2 - 10:30 AM
Meal #3 - 1:30 PM

Pre-Workout Protein Shake 3:00 PM
Workout 3:30 - 5:00 PM
Post-Workout Protein Drink 5:15 PM

Meal #4 - 8:30 AM
Meal #5 - 11:30 AM

What to eat at each meal: Now that you are a bodybuilder your food choices matter allot more than every single normal person you know. Most normal people are not counting the amount of protein, carbohydrates and fat they are consuming with each meal. They are not concerned with where most or for that matter any of their food comes from. Don't care to much about how much its processed and what nutrients are lost during such processing. You as the bodybuilder have to be concerned with all of these variables, yep all right down to the most minute of them. Your foods should be a natural and as leased processed as possible to ensure as much raw nutrient content as possible. The more processed a food source is the more its nutritional value is compromised. As you have read in the previous sections nutrients value is very important in making sure you fulfill your daily and weekly nutrient quota to keep your body is a state of plenty so that it does not have to worry about growth and recovery. Your 1st meal of the day should be one of low glycemic carbs and easily digested protein. One of the best first meals if you are not used to eating early in the morning is to have an apple sliced into 8 pieces with a tablespoon of natural peanut butter on each along with 4-5 chelated amino acid tablets and a cup of coffee. This small meal will get you body used to the ritual of eating upon awakening so that in a few weeks you can graduate to a bowl of oatmeal, eggs, wheat toast and orange juice. After the first meal each subsequent meal should be eaten every 3 to 3.5 hours until training and resumed after that. The biggest part is that you are going to have to adjust to make sure you get your meals in when necessary to keep your body feed properly. Feeding your body properly is the hardest part of becoming a bodybuilder. It is the consistency with getting your meals in day in and day out that will determine if you achieve your goals of adding muscle mass to your physique.

How much to consume at each meal: Figuring out how much your going to consume in the way of macros - Calories, Grams of Protein, Grams of Carbohydrates, and Grams of Fats all come from the calculations that you do at the beginning of each training cycle, when you map you daily and weekly total based on your calculated lean bodyweight. We are not going to make any try to figure out this on your own, use the below online calculator to figure your lean body mass, then use that number to calculate your daily food intake. As you body mass starts to change you will notice yourself becoming leaner, but also your amount of calories consumed rising as well. Your calories will increase because of the shear fact that muscle burns calories and requires nutrients to be sustained where fat does not.

Body Fat Calculator: Click Here

All this may seem very complicated but the use of structured meals planning is so important because it lays down the foundation of when, what and how much to eat.  Remember these simple guidelines:

1. Eat within your first hour of awaking.
2. Eat every 3-3.5 hours.
3. Eat approximately 5 meals and 2 Shakes before and after training.
4. Eat balanced, well-proportioned meals based on your lean body mass.

**Consider these questions to assess your eating:**

- Does my plan allow for me to have adequate time to get all meal in during each day? Make adjustments to allow for all 5 meals and pre/post workout shake.
- Are you nutrient ratios on target for each day and do they meet my weekly totals for all macronutrients.
- Am I gaining body fat or am gaining muscle mass. If your abs are becoming more blurred in the mirror - subtract 100 calories evenly across

all macros each day until weight gain stops. Hold calories at this level until abs are back in focus for at least 3 weeks.
- ❑ Am I loosing weight or feeling tired - add 100 calories evenly across all macros each day until weight loss stops

## **<u>Putting It All Together</u>**

Now that you have all the parts to constructing your own personal meal plan lets start by putting all the pieces together to do just that. We must follow some chronological steps to construct our plan so that it does what we desire, which is to help us add muscle mass to our physique over the course of our training cycles and beyond. All four steps are as follows:

- ❑ Find Lean Body Mass
- ❑ Calculate Protein Needs
- ❑ Calculate all macros - daily & weekly
- ❑ Construct your meals

This sound easy enough, so lets get started.

Find lean Body Mass: We will be using a method developed by the U.S. Navy to help give them a good estimate of the health of it recruits. It is a fairly accurate in its calculation of body mass, and has about a 5% difference +/-. For more accurate measurements of body fat, the use of instruments such as Bioelectric Impedance (BMI - the flow of an electric current through body tissues which can then be used to estimate total body water (TBW), which can be used to estimate fat-free body mass and, by difference with body weight, body fat.) analysis or Hydrostatic Density Testing (under water weighing) is necessary. First you need your age, and weight to input into the calculator. Next we need the following measurements - Neck (Measure the circumference of the subject's neck starting below the larynx, with the tape sloping downward to the front. The subject should avoid flaring their neck outwards.), Waist (Measure the circumference of the subject's waist at a horizontal level around the navel for men, and at the level with the smallest width for women. Ensure that the subject does not pull their stomach inwards to obtain accurate measurements.), Hips (For women only: Measure the circumference of the subject's hips at the largest horizontal measure.) Once you have obtained you measurement simply input your data and record your results.

Ex.

Body Fat Category Fitness

Body Fat Mass      23.2 lbs

Lean Body Mass     128.8 lbs

**Calculate Food Protein Needs:** As you read above we have a recommendation of between 0.8 to 1.2 grams of protein per pound of bodyweight. So our calculation using the above data would look like the following:

128.8 x 1.0 = ~130 grams of Protein per day.

**Calculate all Food Macros - Daily & Weekly:**
Using the 130 grams of protein per day as our guide for this individual into our guidelines of - protein should make up 35% of your daily intake with carbs at 45% and high quality fats rounding everything out at 20%, we come out with the following daily macros.

Calculate Total Food Caloric Daily Intake:

130x4 = 520 Calories

520/0.35 = 1486 Calories Daily Intake

Protein - 130 grams Protein = 520 Calories

Carbohydrates - 167 gram Carbs = 669 Calories

Fats - 33 grams Fats = 297 Calories

----------------------------------------------

= 1486 Food Calories Daily

1486 x 7 = 10,402 Food Calories Weekly

**Construct your Food Meals:** You are going to be eating 5 meals a day so the smart thing would be to first divide your calories up into five equal portions for the day. Then subtract 10% of the calories from 2 meals and give those calories to your first meal of the day and the first meal following your workouts. Your Meal Outline should look as follows:

Meal #1: 327 Calories

Meal #2: 297 Calories

Meal #3: 267 Calories

Meal #4: 327 Calories

Meal #5: 267 Calories

--------------------

Total Food Caloric Intake = 1485 Calories

Now you have your calories per meal, the number of meals and the total calories per day we can start constructing individual meals to fit into our plan. Knowing that we have 2 meals of the same caloric intake and just one a slight bit higher we might want to make these meals using similar foods and vary the ingredients slightly to provide as much variety as possible. With meal #1 being our starter meals of the day its very important we start with a steady energy source so to balance our blood sugar and provide a good source of energy to get us up and going for hours. It would be important to avoid any high glycemic foods and caffeinated drinks until after your second meal of the day. With meal #4 looking like the post workout meal we should focus more on nutrient density for our protein and add in some fibrous carbohydrates to ensure proper digestion and nutrient uptake. That leaves meals #2, #3, and #5 as those left to assign nutrient values. Meals #'s 2 & 3 should build off of meal #1 with the addition of more low glycemic carbs, but lower the amount by the 10% calorie reduction keeping protein and fats the same. Meal #5 is your wrap-up meal of the day and should have little to no low glycemic carbs but replaced with a little more fat and protein, for slower digestion to aide your body while you sleep with amino acids and hormone secretion (Fats help with your hormones). Yeah we know it sound complicated but we give you 2 examples to look at to get a idea of how it should look.

Example Beginning Daily Meal Plan #1

NOTE: **The eating plan was designed for an athlete of 180Lbs beginning bodybuilder college student. So it is a good example for anyone looking for a starting point.**

## Beginning 12 Week Training Cycle: BWT 181 Lbs. Ending BWT 192 Lbs.
## Calculated Totals:

- Body Fat Category Athletes
- Body Fat Mass 14.0 lbs
- Lean Body Mass 166.0 lbs

166.0 x 1.2 = ~199 grams of Protein per day.

Protein - 199 grams Protein = 796 Calories
Carbohydrates - 256 gram Carbs = 1026 Calories
Fats - 51 grams Fats = 455 Calories
-----------------------------------------------
= 2277 Food Calories Per Day

## Actual Meal Schedule and Daily Totals

| 5 Day Basic Bodybuilding Meal Plan |
| --- |

|  | Calories | Protein* | Carbs* | Fats* |
| --- | --- | --- | --- | --- |
| Meal #1 - 7:00AM | | | | |
| 2 Whole xLarge Eggs 1 xLarge Egg White | 186 | 19g | 1g | 11g |
| 1 Cup Oatmeal Cooked (Old Fashion) | 145 | 6g | 25g | 2g |
| 1 Cup 2% Milk | 122 | 8g | 11g | 5g |
| 1 Medium Banana | 105 | 1g | 27g | 0g |
|  | | | | |
| Meal #2 - 9:30AM | | | | |
| 2 Scoops Whey Protein* | 170 | 44g | 2g | <1g |
| 1 oz. Mixed Nuts | 175 | 5g | 6g | 16g |
|  | | | | |
| Meal #3 - 12:30PM | | | | |
| 2 Slices Whole Wheat Bread | 120 | 8g | 22g | 1g |
| 1/2 large (About 6 oz. yield after cooking, bone and skin removed) Roasted Skinless Chicken Breast | 161 | 30g | 0g | 3g |
| 2 Cups Salad Mix | 44 | 3g | 8g | 0g |
| 1 tbsp of Fat Free Mayo/Salad Dressing (Miracle Whip Light) | 11/37 | 0g/0g | 0g/0g | 0g/3.5g |

| 1 Cup Unsweetened Apple Sauce (Motts) | 100 | 0g | 28g | 0g |
|---|---|---|---|---|
| | | | | |
| **Pre-Workout Shake 3:00PM (30 Minutes Before)** | | | | |
| 1.5 Scoop Whey Protein Isolate | 130 | 30g | 1.5g | 0g |
| 10 Grams (~1 Tablespoon) Now Sports Dextrose Powder | 35 | 0g | 9g | 0g |
| 3-5 Grams Creatine Monohydrate | 0 | 0g | 0g | 0g |
| 5 Grams (¾ Teaspoon) L-Citrulline | 0 | 0g | 0g | 0g |
| 1 Large Orange | 86 | 2g | 22g | 0g |
| | | | | |
| **Post-Workout Shake 5:00PM (Wihtin 30 Minutes After)** | | | | |
| 2 Scoop Whey Protein Isolate | 170 | 42g | 2g | <1g |
| 5 (~ 1 Teaspoon) Grams Creatine Monohydrate | 0 | 0g | 0g | 0g |
| 5 (~ 1 Teaspoon) Grams Glutamine | 0 | 0g | 0g | 0g |
| 1 Medium Banana | 105 | 1g | 27g | 0g |
| | | | | |
| **Meal #4 7:30PM** | | | | |
| Ground Beef, | 230 | 36g | 0g | 9g |

| | | | | |
|---|---|---|---|---|
| 95% Lean Meat (6 0z Raw Meat) | | | | |
| 1 Cups Brown Rice - Cooked | 216 | 5g | 45g | 4g |
| 1 Cup Mixed Vegetables - Frozen | 118 | 5g | 24g | 0.2g |
| ½ Cup Coleslaw | 41 | 1g | 7.5g | 1.6g |
| 2 tbsp Kraft Free Fat Free Ranch Dressing | 48 | 0g | 11g | 0.5g |
| 1 Can Diet Soda 12 oz (Diet Coke) | 4 | 0g | 0g | 0g |
| | | | | |
| Meal #5 10:30PM | | | | |
| 1 Scoop Casein Protein* | 120 | 23g | 4g | 1g |
| 1 Cup 2% Milk | 122 | 8g | 11g | 5g |
| 2 tbsp Natural Chunky Peanut Butter | 200 | 8g | 6g | 16g |
| | | | | |
| **TOTALS** | **2464 Calories From Food** | **210.0g Pro.** | **234.5g Carbs** | **78.8g Fat** |
| | **2990 Calories Including Pre/Post Meals** | **285.0g Pro.** | **296g Carbs** | **78.8g Fat** |

This eating plan is not meant for those with blood sugar disorders because its carbohydrate demands are very high and will add stress to the hardest raining athletes system. The plan should be followed for periods of 6-8 weeks when you are building toward competition and need those extra calories and higher than normal nutrient content. Calories will vary slightly from actual total by ~5%.

## Example Advanced Daily Meal Plan #2

NOTE: **The eating plan was designed for an athlete of 220Lbs competitive bodybuilding. So it is a good example for anyone looking for a starting point that has been working toward competition.**

**Beginning 12 Week Training Cycle: BWT 222 Lbs. Ending BWT 236 Lbs.**
**Calculated Total:**

- Body Fat Category Athletes
- Body Fat Mass 16.2 lbs
- Lean Body Mass 203.8 lbs

203.8 x 1.2 = ~245 grams of Protein per day.

Protein - 245 grams Protein = 980 Calories
Carbohydrates - 315 gram Carbs = 1260 Calories
Fats - 62 grams Fats = 560 Calories
-----------------------------------------------
= 2800 Food Calories Per Day

## Actual Meal Schedule and Daily Totals

| 5 Day Basic Bodybuilding Meal Plan | | | | |
|---|---|---|---|---|
| | Calories | Protein* | Carbs* | Fats* |
| Meal #1 - 7:00AM | | | | |
| 4 Whole xLarge Eggs Scrambled | 340 | 29g | 2g | 22.8g |

| | | | | |
|---|---|---|---|---|
| 1 Cup Oatmeal Cooked (Old Fashion) | 145 | 6g | 25g | 2g |
| 1 Cup 2% Milk | 122 | 8g | 11g | 5g |
| 1 Medium Banana | 105 | 1g | 27g | 0g |
| | | | | |
| **Meal #2 - 9:30AM** | | | | |
| 1 6.5oz Can Water Pack Tuna | 194 | 42.6g | 0g | 1g |
| 2 Slices of Whole Wheat Bread | 120 | 8g | 22g | 1g |
| 1 Medium Tomato Diced | 22 | 1g | 5g | 0g |
| 2 tbsp Banquet Light Mayonnaise | 20 | 0g | 4g | 0g |
| 1 Cup Chopped Lettuces | 8 | .5g | 2g | 0g |
| 1 4oz. Cup Unsweetened Apple Sauce | 50 | 0g | 13g | 0g |
| | | | | |
| **Meal #3 - 12:00PM** | | | | |
| 8 oz Roasted Skinless Chicken Breast | 296 | 45g | 0g | 12g |
| 1.5 Cups White Rice | 363 | 6g | 80g | 1g |
| 1 Cup Mix Frozen Vegetable | 75 | 3g | 16g | 0g |

| | | | | |
|---|---|---|---|---|
| Steamed (Birdseye) | | | | |
| 1 Cup Coffee & Low cal Sweetener | 2 | 0g | 0g | 0g |
| | | | | |
| **Preworkout Shake 2:30PM (30 Minutes Before)** | | | | |
| 2 Scoop Whey Protein Isolate | 170 | 42g | 2g | <1g |
| 10 Grams (~1 tbsp) Now Sports Dextrose Powder | 35 | 0g | 9g | 0g |
| 5-8 Grams Creatine Monohydrate | 0 | 0g | 0g | 0g |
| 5 Grams (¾ Teaspoon) L-Citrulline | 0 | 0g | 0g | 0g |
| | | | | |
| **Postworkout Shake 4:30PM (Wihtin 30 Minutes After)** | | | | |
| 2 Scoop Whey Protein Isolate | 170 | 42g | 2g | <1g |
| 5 (~ 1 tsp) Grams Creatine Monohydrate | 0 | 0g | 0g | 0g |
| 10 (~ 2 tsp) Grams Glutamine | 0 | 0g | 0g | 0g |
| 1 Medium Banana | 105 | 1g | 27g | 0g |
| | | | | |
| **Meal #4 7:00PM** | | | | |
| 8 oz Roasted | 296 | 45g | 0g | 12g |

| | | | | |
|---|---|---|---|---|
| Skinless Chicken Breast | | | | |
| 1.5 Cups Brown Rice - Cooked | 216 | 5g | 45g | 4g |
| 1 Cup Mixed Vegetables - Frozen | 118 | 5g | 24g | 0.2g |
| 1 Cup Coleslaw (Shredded Cabbage, Carrots, Beets) | 83 | 2g | 15g | 2g |
| 2 tbsp Kraft Free Fat Free Ranch Dressing | 48 | 0g | 11g | 0.5g |
| 1 Can Diet Soda 12 oz (Diet Coke) | 4 | 0g | 0g | 0g |
| | | | | |
| Meal #5 10:00PM | | | | |
| 3 xLarge Eggs Boiled | 267 | 22g | 2g | 18g |
| 1 Cup Oatmeal Cooked (Old Fashion) | 145 | 6g | 25g | 2g |
| 1 Cup 2% Milk | 122 | 8g | 11g | 5g |
| 2 tbsp Natural Chunky Peanut Butter | 200 | 8g | 6g | 16g |
| | | | | |
| **TOTALS** | **3361 Calories From Food** | **251.1.0g Pro.** | **334.0g Carbs** | **105.0g Fat** |

| | 3841 Calories Including Pre/Post Meals | 336.1g Pro. | 374.0g Carbs | 105.8g Fat |
| --- | --- | --- | --- | --- |
| This eating plan is not meant for those with blood sugar disorders because its carbohydrate demands are very high and will add stress to the hardest raining athletes system. The plan should be followed for periods of 6-12 weeks when you are building toward competition and need those extra calories and higher than normal nutrient content. Calories will vary slightly from actual total by ~5%. | | | | |

**Tips and Tricks for building your plan:** The very first thing we want you to do before anything is to take 4 photo of your physique as follows: front, both sides, and back. These should be used to judge your appearance on a bi-weekly basis. What you can see by these 2 plans is that they differ from the statistical measures derived from the body fat measurement. Each meal plan was adjusted up until each athlete stop loosing weight, stabilized, then start to add weight at a slow but steady rate. Lets get this out right here and now - **THERE IS NO APP., NO PLAN OF ANY KIND THAT IS CORRECT AND FULLY FUNCTIONAL AT INITIATION! NONE!** It doesn't matter who wrote it or so-called credentials the supposed Guru touts is going to make that untrue. Always adjust your up or down after 14 days depending on what going on with your body weight, physical appearance, and energy levels. Use the scale below to determine your adjustments:

Loosing Bodyweight: If your loosing weight more than 3 Lbs. a week - which signals some muscle lose up your calories by 5-10% per day which may mean just adding say 2tblspns of peanut butter to a meal (yeah it can sometimes be that simple). If you're loosing only 1-2 Lbs. a week check your measurement and look at your physique photos and you will see a lost in body fat and a slight gain in muscle mass. No adjustment necessary.

Gaining Weight to fast: If you are gaining more than 2 pounds a week you are gaining too much bodyweight per week. Much of the body mass you're putting on is not muscle mass. Lower your daily calories by 100 calories a day for the next 2 weeks and note the weight gain on the second week. If it has lowered to around 2 pounds you have stabilized for now and revisit this at the end of the next 2 weeks, if 2 Lbs. is still there mean you don't require any other adjustments.

Feeling Tired after each Meal: Ad more fibrous carbohydrates to you 2 post workout meals. These carbs keep your metabolism moving which is very critical to your energy levels.

Not loosing Weight but loosing Strength: If your loosing strength over 2 weeks you need to add 10% more protein to your diet to help feed your muscles. This may also be correlated with loosing bodyweight.

Final Tip: Do not be scared of doing your own eating plan. Paying someone for one of his or her retread meal plans is a complete waste of your money. They don't know your eating history or for that matter your medical history. Take the time, about a week and design your own, it will work allot better for you and won't cost you 1 thin dime. Good luck and don't hesitate to do this yourself.

# Chapter 7 Bodybuilding Lifestyle

## It's About the Work

Now that you have chosen one of the most rewarding sport occupations on the planet you should feel very good 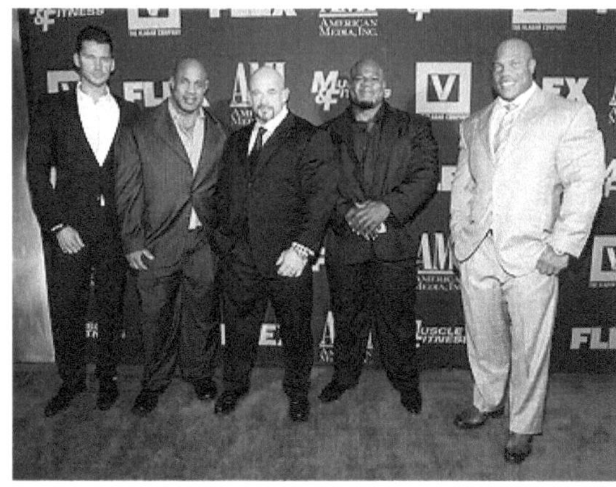 about yourself. Bodybuilding is way more than just lifting weights and eating good food, it offers you they way to transform your whole way of life. Being a success in bodybuilding requires you to adopt a different way of thinking and acting. Unlike becoming say a teacher, dentist or even a doctor, all great occupations in their own right none require you to adopt a new way of living that is very contrary from the norm. Matter of fact you can be all those occupations listed and adding bodybuilding on to them would make you even more successful than you were before. Why am I touting the effects of bodybuilding so much is that to be successful you are going to have to learn 4 things right from the get go:

- ❑ **You must be consistent:** Consistency is your workouts and nutritional habits are the most crucial traits that must be formed in the pursuit of the bodybuilding physique. Workouts and meals must only be missed due to sickness and life threatening emergencies.

- **You must plan out your time:** You have heard the phrase if you don't plan than you plan to loose, well in bodybuilding that is not just a saying it is the mantra. If you don't plan than will definitely loose. As bodybuilding legend Arnold Schwarzenegger has said "You can have the best ship in the world, but without a plan you are going to just sail around the seas forever". Translation - No plan, No Success!

- **You must the resolve to finish:** Finishing is building the trait of always doing the job to completion no matter what. Stopping a set of heavy squats on the 3rd rep when you can do 3 more does you NO good toward reaching your goals. You must be able to accept the grind and push forward to the end of each set, and relish in the small victories of finishing.

- **You must be able to accept failure:** One of the best lessons in bodybuilding is that of failure. You learn allot more in failure than you will ever learn in winning. Failure teaches you that even if you do everything right you still may not win on that given day. Each time you get up, dust your self off and go back at it your moving your moving your self forward towards your goals. This trait along with consistency will take you to new height in just about every walk of your life when applied. Never fear failure, learn from it and try again.

Yeah we can hear it now from people in other sports saying we have those things also, but in reality you don't. You have an on season and a off season. Bodybuilding is an always-on sport, contests preparation or not. Your inconsistency in any area of your training or diet will set you back weeks maybe months. Other sports don't have this. Failure to plan is the same; no plan and you can kiss off winning, as genetics in bodybuilding will only get you to the stage not the winner's circle.

All these aspects, the consistency, the planning, and the acceptance of failure are so of the most important characteristics of success in just about every successful person past present and future. Many a professional, and Amateur bodybuilders are some very good businessmen and women as these are the traits of success. So when you are lamenting the grid of the training and eating you are forming habits that transfer into any and all professions current or future. It all about the work!

## The Giving Way

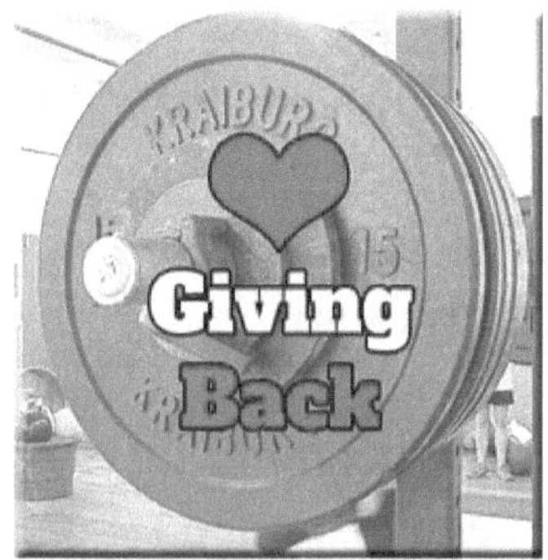


Bodybuilding at time is probably the most narcissistic sports one can imagine, it requires self focus on a 24 hr. basis. This one of the very reasons most bodybuilders are looked upon as self-centered and egotistical people. The truth about most of us bodybuilders is quite the opposite. Most give of themselves in many different ways and allot of the time to their own

88

determent almost. We here at MuscleSports.com give of our time explaining exercise concepts and different nutrition or supplement information to just about any one that ask. It just what you do if you care about the sport or business your in. Now I am not saying that there aren't times when you might not get your question answered or have that selfie taken, but for the most part the bodybuilding community is a very friendly and giving place of advice and information on a variety of related subjects.

You as an up and coming bodybuilder should strive to do the same as those of the past and give back what you have learned. In today technological age of social media have way more outlets to do this than in past generations. Starting a blog, website, **Facebook** or **Twitter** page so be one of your main forms of getting your name out and self marketing. People like to know of those like them who have been there and are now achieving some of their goals. Keeping such an online journal also makes you more memorable and exposes you to finding more sponsorships and being able to reach more people with your message. Remember if you give in a honest and open way you'll receive 10 times more positive feedback than if you try to over market and monetize everything you want to convey to people.

# <u>Never Stop Learning</u>

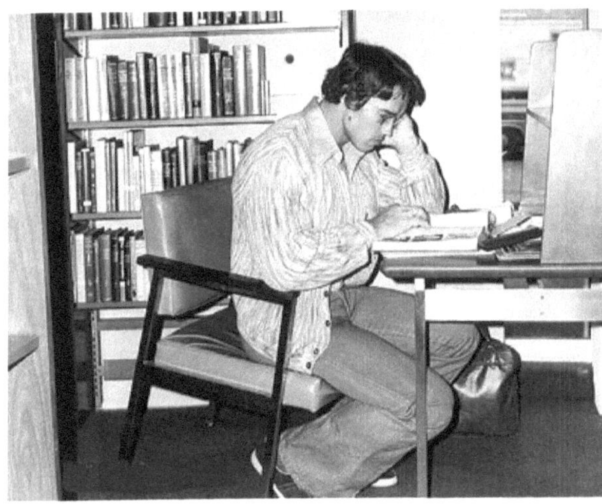

The last thing we want to say to you as aspiring is to never stop learning. We mean real educated learning. We are not talking about the stuff you'll get from some yahoo on Youtube blowing smoke out his ass about some new supplement or technique that's going to put 50 pounds on your bench in one week. The main question that you have to ask these people consist of just 4 little words:

## <u>HOW DO YOU KNOW?</u>

Its four simple words that if they have a very good reason why then you may want to look into their claim. More than likely though, they will come back with even more BS of a sales pitch.

We are talking about taking class offered at your local community college on business, nutrition, sociology and things of that nature. One of the riches and most educated billionaires in the world Bill Gates reads and studies psychology. His business isn't based on the mind of people but knowing how people think can help his business. Knowing a little more about sociology could help your personal training business down the line or improve social skills in professional setting. Never stop learning about life because **"The More You Know, The Less Likely Your to Lose"**.

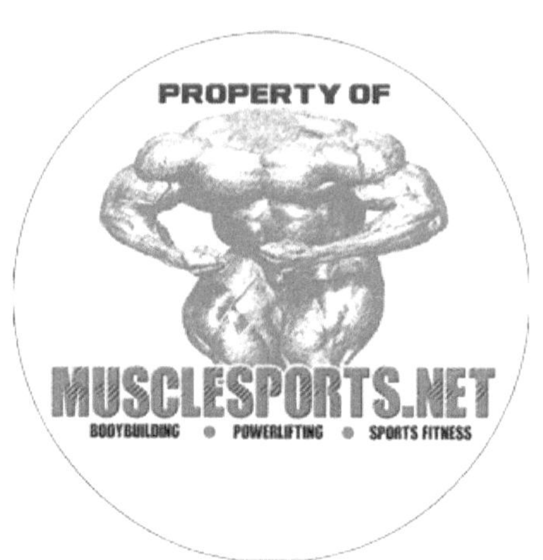


# Conclusion

In conclusion this has been a fun book to write. I was asked to write this book about 2 years ago but didn't because I look out there and saw allot of other books and though, eh the topic is very much covered. Then the same friend told me that the way we teach has lasted with him for the last 10 years and up to today. The book holds on to the basic truths of what bodybuilding is all about. Bodybuilding isn't about trying to lift 700 Lbs. in the bench (it can get you there), its about muscle control, movement and function on the training front. We relied on sound steady nutritional concepts that rely on food more than supplements. When it comes to nutrition we cut it short as that is a concept for another book. It was fun talking about the guys of the 40's and 50's who pioneered physique training like John Grimek and Steve Reeves. Going into the 60's and 70's, which form the basis of what bodybuilding training is even by today's machine oriented training. All of today's machines just try to mimic the exercises of the past. The manual is informative, concise in its information. This style and form of training is timeless and will last all though who follow it for their entire lives without alteration or adjustment.

93

**Thank You**

DL.

# <u>References</u>:


## Protein – Which is Best?
J Sports Sci Med. 2004 Sep; 3(3): 118–130.
Published online 2004 Sep 1.
https://www.ncbi.nlm.nih.gov/pmc/articles/PMC3905294/

## Glycemic Index
The University of Sydney
http://www.glycemicindex.com/

## Body Fat Calculator
Calculators.net
https://www.calculator.net/body-fat-calculator.html

## Grocery Shopping List
Shopping List
http://www.musclesports.net/articles/Nutrition/plist.html

## Printable Workout Logs
Workout Logs
http://www.musclesports.net/articles/Bodybuilding/WorkLog.htm